expecting Adam

Also by Martha Beck

Breaking Point

expecting Adam

A True Story of Birth, Transformation & Unconditional Love

MARTHA BECK

PIATKUS

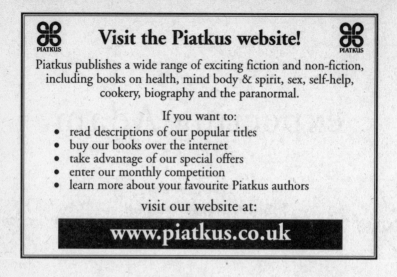

Grateful acknowledgement is made to Broadway Books, a division of Random House, for permission to reprint an extract from *The Illuminated Rumi* by Coleman Barks and Michael Green.

First published in the United States by Times Books

Published in the UK in 2000 by
Judy Piatkus (Publishers) Ltd
5 Windmill Street
London W1T 2JA
e-mail: info@piatkus.co.uk

Reprinted 2000
This edition first published 2001

The moral rights of the author have been asserted

*A catalogue record for this book is available
from the British Library*

ISBN 0 7499 2077 7

Printed and bound in Great Britain by
Mackays of Chatham PLC, Chatham, Kent

For my boy

EXPECTING
ADAM

1

⮎ This happened when Adam was about three years old.

I was sitting in a small apartment with a woman I had barely met, talking to her about her life. I'll call her Mrs. Ross, because it isn't her name. I had been doing similar interviews for months, collecting data for my Ph.D. dissertation. Mrs. Ross was a scrawny forty-five-year-old with a master's degree in art history and a job as an elementary school janitor. I was taking notes, considering what this woman's experience had to teach about the real-world value of the more refined academic fields, when she suddenly stopped talking.

There was a moment of silence, and then I looked up and said, "Yes?" in a helpful voice, which was normally enough to keep an interview rolling. But Mrs. Ross wasn't acting normal. She had been sitting on a straight-backed wooden chair, both feet set firmly on the floor and her hands resting primly on her knees. Now she was curled into an almost fetal position, forearms crushed between the tops of her thighs and her chest, her eyes tightly closed.

I became alarmed. "Are you all right?" I said, trying to sound politely but not overly curious.

Mrs. Ross waved a hand at me. "I can't . . . quite . . . make it out," she said.

I just stared at her.

"Usually," she gasped, her eyelids clamping down tighter, "usually I can tell which side of the veil it's coming from . . . that's usually the first thing I can tell . . . but this time I . . . can't."

"Uh-huh," I said cautiously, glancing toward the door, wondering if I could get to it before Mrs. Ross leapt upon me like a mad dog.

"It's like . . . he's not really on one side of the veil or the other . . . maybe he's on *both*." She shook her head, troubled. "At least I know it's a he."

3

"Uh, Mrs. Ross," I said, gathering my notes together for a quick exit.

At this point Mrs. Ross's eyes flew open wide, fixing me with a bloodshot stare.

"You know who it is!" she said in a low, accusing voice. "You know who it is, but you're blocking!"

At this point my curiosity began to get the better of me. "I know who?" I said.

"That's right!" Mrs. Ross uncurled a little. "You see, I have this . . . well, it's a gift." She sounded as though she wasn't quite sure Santa had gotten her letters.

"Gift?" I repeated.

She nodded. "I get messages for people." She sighed and sat up. "There was a point in my life when I stopped talking about it, you know, because it's very embarrassing."

"Oh," I said.

"And then, you know," Mrs. Ross continued, "I began to lose it. It was getting fainter, and sometimes the spirits would be angry at me, because I wouldn't help them get through to people."

At this moment, I swear to God, a large green parrot walked out of Mrs. Ross's small kitchen and into the living room. It paced slowly across the carpet, peered at me suspiciously with one flinty eye, then proceeded on foot up the leg of Mrs. Ross's chair and onto her shoulder. She's a witch, I thought. I'm sitting here talking to a genuine witch. The parrot was obviously a familiar. I would have been willing to bet it was her husband.

Mrs. Ross kept talking, stroking the bird absentmindedly. "So I promised God that I would always deliver the messages as soon as I got them. No matter what."

"No kidding." I said this without any sarcasm. That's how much I had changed. Four years earlier I would have dismissed Mrs. Ross and her "gift" immediately. Back then I had known exactly how the world worked. Back then I had been sure of my own intellect, sure of the primacy of Reason, sure that, given enough time and training, I could control my destiny. That was before Adam. But now it was four years later, and Adam was at home with the baby-sitter, and I had learned a lot about how much I had to learn. So I sat still and waited for Mrs. Ross to go on. She did.

"The messages are usually from the other side of the veil—I mean, from the spirit world," she said. "Sometimes they're from living people who are far away and need to get a message through immediately. But that's always the first thing I can tell—which side of the veil the message is coming from." Her brow furrowed. "And this time, I can't tell."

By now, I admit it, I was hooked. I wanted my message.

"Just relax," I suggested helpfully.

Mrs. Ross shot me a glance that would have pierced steel, a glance designed to shove me off her turf.

"Or not," I said.

"We should pray," whispered Mrs. Ross.

"Uh, okeydokey," I responded. I mean, what would you have done?

So Mrs. Ross and I bowed our heads, and I drew a deep breath and relaxed for just a second, and then her head snapped up like a Pez dispenser and she said, "All right, you stopped blocking. It's your son."

"My son?" Even after everything that had already happened, this surprised me. I had been hoping the message would be from my guardian angel, or perhaps a stray ancestor with an interest in my career.

"You have a son who's halfway between worlds," stated Mrs. Ross.

I felt the hair go up on my arms. You see, no matter how much evidence you have, over time you tend to block out the experiences that aren't "normal." Who wants to turn into a Mrs. Ross, blurting out gibberish about spirits and veils? How much of that sort of conversation are you allowed before people stop inviting you to parties, and you end up pushing a mop in an elementary school?

"Well," I said to Mrs. Ross, "maybe I do have a son . . . uh . . . like that."

She gave me a withering look. "You do," she said flatly. "And he wants me to give you a message." The parrot nibbled tenderly on her ear.

By now my whole body was bristling with a strange electricity. The sensation had become familiar to me over the past few years, yet it was always a surprise. At least I kept my mouth shut.

Mrs. Ross closed her eyes again, gently this time. "He says that he's been watching you very closely from both sides of the veil."

The veil again.

"He says that you shouldn't be so worried. He says you'll never be hurt as much by being open as you have been hurt by remaining closed."

She opened her eyes, scratched the parrot's head, and smiled. She didn't look like a witch at all anymore.

"That's it?" I said.

Mrs. Ross nodded, smiling.

I didn't return the smile. "What the heck is that supposed to mean?"

She shrugged. "Beats me."

"Oh, come on," I pleaded. "There's got to be more. Ask him." This is not the way I was taught to behave at Harvard.

"I don't ask questions," she said. "I just deliver messages. Like Western Union. What the messages mean is none of my business."

And that was all she had to say.

After a pathetic attempt to pretend I was still conducting an interview, I raced home to confront Adam. He was in his crib, asleep. He was about half the size of a normal three-year-old, had barely learned to walk, and had never spoken an intelligible word. I reached down and poked him in the tummy, and he woke up with his usual jolly grin on his face.

I looked into his small, slanted eyes. "Adam," I said seriously. "You've got to tell me. Are you sending me messages through Mrs. Ross?"

His smile broadened. That was all. And he hasn't said a thing about it since.

⮑ So here I am, still wondering what the hell happened that day, wondering whether Mrs. Ross was really channeling my three-year-old, wondering what he meant. I wonder a lot of things, since Adam came along. I wonder about all the strange and beautiful and terrible things that accompanied him into my life. My husband, John, knows about my wondering—shares it, in fact, since his life, too, was changed when we were expecting Adam. But when I wasn't talking to John, I learned to keep it all to myself. I learned to ignore the miraculous in my life, to pretend it didn't exist, to tell lies in order to be believed. In short, I kept myself closed.

This has not been easy. It is difficult *not* to tell people when one of your interview subjects turns out to be Parrot Woman. The strangeness, the curiosity, the wonder keeps pushing outward, begging to be communicated, needing air and company. On many occasions, I have tried to talk about Adam without letting on that I actually believed in everything that happened to me. I have written this book twice already, both times as a novel, to wit: "This is the story of two driven Harvard academics who found out in midpregnancy that their unborn son would be retarded. To their own surprise and the horrified dismay of the university community, the couple ignored the abundant means, motive, and opportunity to obtain a therapeutic abortion. They decided to allow their baby to be born. What they did not realize is that they themselves were the ones who would be 'born,' infants in a new world where magic is commonplace, Harvard professors are the slow learners, and retarded babies are the master teachers."

You see, by calling it a novel, I could tell the story without putting myself in danger from skeptics, scientists, and intellectuals. "Fiction!" I would assure them. "Made it all up! Not a word of truth in it!" Then they would all go away and leave me alone, and perhaps a few sturdy souls would be willing to believe me, and I could open up in safety to them.

It hasn't worked out that way. The editors and agents and writers I respect most have always come back, after reading my "novel," with the same question: "Excuse me, but how much of this is fiction?" And I would hem and haw a bit before admitting that aside from making John and myself sound much better-looking than we are, I didn't fictionalize anything. It's all true, I would say. Then I would sink into my chair five or six inches and wait for them to call security.

So far, that hasn't happened. It has been five years since Mrs. Ross reared back against her parrot and delivered Adam's message, and in all that time my favorite people have continually repeated his advice. Open up, they say. It will feel better than remaining closed.

I am none too sure about this. I am very much afraid of being caught in the firestorms of controversy over abortion, genetic engineering, medical ethics. It worries me to think that I will be lumped together with the right-to-lifers, not to mention every New Age crystal kisser who ever claimed to see an angel in the clouds over Sedona. I am reluctant to wave good-bye to my rationalist credibility. Nevertheless, the story will not stop unfolding, and it will not stop asking me to tell it. I have resisted it for what feels like a very long time, hoping it would back off and disappear. But it hasn't.

So, Mrs. Ross, wherever you are, thank you for delivering my son's message. After all these years, I've finally decided to listen.

2

John and I disagree about the precise moment we lost control of our lives. He thinks it was the car accident in New Hampshire. I say it was two weeks before that, when Adam was conceived. Either way, it was sometime in September of 1987, which ever since has been known in our family history as the month It All Went to Hell.

We had just returned to Cambridge from a summer in Tokyo, where John had been doing research for a Ph.D. dissertation on the Japanese employment system. We were dazed with jet lag, which is bad enough for an adult crossing fourteen time zones but turns into an epic struggle when you're traveling with a toddler. Our eighteen-month-old daughter, Katie, was still operating on Japanese time, babbling and playing through the Boston nights while John and I took turns trying to sleep. By the time the sun showed up and Katie closed her maddeningly bright little eyes, we would have to stumble off, haggard and woozy, to deal with the welter of logistical tasks involved in preparing to go to Harvard.

Again.

There are some things you have to understand about Harvard. First of all, John and I both grew up there. I'm not talking about childhood. I mean later on, when all our adult thoughts and expectations were being programmed. As for childhood, we both spent that in the same small town in Utah, a state that doesn't register as part of the known universe to anyone in the Ivy League. (One of my professors once told me he'd just returned from my region of the country. I said, "Oh really? Where?" He said, "Iowa." And he meant it.) As a matter of fact, this writing marks the first time I've actually admitted in public that I am a child of the lovely Beehive State. Harvard trained me to believe that this is like admitting to a history of mental illness or shoplifting. It would have bought me much more credibility if I'd been able to claim that I'd been reared by wolves.

9

The point is that neither John nor I relied on anything that happened to us before Harvard to guide our behavior once we got there. John arrived when he was eighteen, and I showed up two years later, in 1980, aged seventeen. We had known each other in high school, but only vaguely; by the time we really got acquainted, we'd both managed to become thoroughly Harvardized. We had a lot in common: the dirty secret of our western public school past, an intense drive to succeed, a longing to fit in. We worked like demons, taking heavy loads of the most difficult classes we could find, so that when we got the phone call saying that the admissions department had just realized its glaring mistake in accepting us, we'd have a fighting chance of remaining enrolled. As a result, we did well academically and ended up going to Harvard over and over again, like addicts. We both applied to combined master's and Ph.D. programs before we'd even graduated from the college. John pursued his passionate study of Asia, while I focused on the sociology of gender. By September of 1987 we had been Harvard students for almost a third of our lives, and we weren't anywhere near finished.

You might assume from all this that John and I found Harvard pleasant. Oh, how wrong you would be. Actually, I don't know if I ever met anyone at Harvard who found it pleasant. It seems to me (although I may well be projecting) that all the people there scurry anxiously from one achievement to another, casting wary glances over their shoulders, never quite sure that they've managed to throw failure off their scent. To me, being a student there was heady, exciting, even thrilling, but these sensations came laced with heavy doses of fear and misery. It was like having lunch with a brilliant, learned, witty celebrity who liked to lean across the table at unpredictable intervals and slap me in the mouth—hard. Was it interesting? Very. Stimulating? In more ways than one. Pleasant? I don't think so.

And so, no matter how many times we did them, the muddle of small tasks surrounding each semester's registration always threw John and me into jittering anxiety that made us snap at each other and break things accidentally. Of course, neither of us would have confessed this under torture, not even to each other. We had been trained against it. At

Harvard, the appearance of confidence is essential to social survival. Without it, you're like the wounded animal in the herd, attracting the full attention of predators and the disdain of most potential mates. (It was only after John and I fell in love, during finals the first semester of his senior year at Harvard, that I worked up the courage to tell him how scared I was of failing. He had confessed to similar feelings. This interchange was enough to bond us forever. It was more intimate than sex.)

Now John was in the third year of his doctoral program, and no one would have guessed that he'd ever had a moment of lagging confidence. He appeared sublimely self-assured despite the fact that not only was he finishing his degree (which would have been stressful in itself) but he had also jumped at an opportunity to work as a management consultant. The firm that hired him had a branch in Boston and was opening a new one in Singapore. John's job involved commuting from New England to Southeast Asia every two weeks during the upcoming year. This would be a tricky thing to pull off without ruffling various feathers at Harvard, so John was even more nervous than usual. Of course, no one knew this except me, and I was just guessing.

To say that hiding my fears did not come naturally to me is to make a profound understatement. I had a tendency to babble hysterically and blink a lot whenever I dealt with Harvard. At least I'd learned to fake self-confidence, probably as well as the next graduate student. I was very deliberate about this. Before I went on the campus for any reason, I would consciously call up a portion of my personality I call Fang. I would focus very hard on being Fang, until I could squash down every thought or feeling that wasn't part of her. Fang fit in beautifully at Harvard. She was fearless, aggressive, sardonic, voraciously competitive. She never ate entire pound bags of M & M's or sat with her feet in the bathroom sink, crying, the way I was wont to do after a hard day's lunch with the slapping celebrity. I had relied on Fang since my freshman year, and she had served me well. But for some reason, in the fall of 1987 I couldn't quite get her revved up. It wasn't just the jet lag, the fatigue, the change of climate. Even then, when Adam was almost entirely unassembled, I knew it was something more.

I remember the very moment I felt the life controls slip out of my fingers. It was the first time since our return from Tokyo that Katie actually dozed off before sunrise. John and I were both trying, unsuccessfully, to fall asleep ourselves. We stared fitfully at the ceiling, the walls, the window that looked out over Harvard Square, thinking about the dangers that awaited us at daybreak. And then, somewhere toward morning, we rolled over simultaneously, met in the center of our queen-size futon, and began to grope for comfort in each other's arms. I told myself it was a bad idea. I told myself I'd better get some rest while Katie was napping. I told these things to John, too. He agreed with me. And then, of course, we went right ahead with it.

In Japan I had seen a style of puppet theater called Bunraku, where the puppeteers stand right onstage, moving these elegant dolls around without the slightest pretense of invisibility. The puppeteers are so skillful that you actually forget they're on the stage, even though there are often three of them to each puppet. After a few minutes, you'd swear the puppets were moving themselves. That night in our apartment, I kept expecting to see two teams of Bunraku masters standing behind John and me, pulling levers in our heads, sculpting every move we made. I could feel them. And without letting it anywhere near my conscious mind, I knew—I *knew*—that I was in the process of getting pregnant, and that it was exactly what I wanted to do.

Mind you, this was insane. I didn't have time to be pregnant. I was well aware of this, because I (or at least Fang) was the kind of person who made elaborate and detailed plans for my life several years in advance. I am not exaggerating here. You could always tell where I'd been by following the trail of paper scraps with time grids and to-do lists scribbled on them. I was the unofficial mascot of the Franklin Dayplanner people, my schedule fixed in fifteen-minute intervals for years to come. That September was the worst possible time for me to exercise my fertility option. I was taking a full load of classes, teaching sections for a course in Caribbean society, and planning to be Katie's single parent when John was in Asia. The very last thing I could afford to do was bear live young again. For one thing, during my first go-round, pregnancy had made me feel only slightly better than the Ebola virus would have. For another thing, I had to guard my reputation as a scholar.

I understand that nowadays there are enough young parents in the Graduate School of Arts and Sciences to support a graduate student "parenting center," but this was not true when I was young and fruitful of loin. Back then, even the potential for motherhood was most definitely a blot on the credibility of female students and staff. I had several friends who obtained abortions when accidental pregnancies threatened to scuttle their academic progress. One woman I knew decided, with her husband, to abort a planned pregnancy when a crucial three-day exam was scheduled near her due date. I don't know whether she even asked if the exam could be rescheduled. That sort of thing simply wasn't done—especially not for "personal reasons."

It often seemed to me that success at Harvard depended on being willing to put "personal reasons" so low on one's priority list that they dropped right off the bottom. John and I had learned this lesson the hard way. For instance, a year and a half before It All Went to Hell, when John was going through the first year of the Harvard Business School curriculum (en route to his Ph.D. in organizational behavior), he missed a day of class taking me to the hospital and Lamaze-coaching me through Katie's birth. The next day, when he went back to the Business School after forty-eight hours without sleep, he received a tongue-lashing that made him wake up in a cold sweat for months afterward. It was delivered in front of the eighty-nine other students in the class by one of his professors, a world-renowned economic theorist I will call Stinky.

"You are a disgrace to this institution," ranted Stinky, while John's classmates sat looking uncomfortably at the floor. "You will never succeed in business, scholarship, or anything else. You have set a bad example for this entire section, and I intend to hold you personally responsible for the poor performance of any student in this room."

When John mumbled that he had wanted to see his child's birth, the professor sneered, said, "You probably think that's a good excuse," and suggested that John should fail out of the class then and there.

You've got to understand that we took this very seriously. I had been away from Harvard for years before I began to realize that not everyone in the United States would agree with Stinky. What amazes me now is that, at the time, both John and I assumed that everyone in the Real World (read: anywhere but Utah) shared Stinky's opinions. So you can see why getting pregnant again on the very eve of an academic year was not part of my conscious master plan, and why that night on our futon felt so trancelike and alien to me. It was like swimming against a riptide: you think you're making lots of progress as you slap away at the water, not even feeling the current, because it is so large and powerful that you aren't able to comprehend it. Then you look at the shore and realize you are in a place you never intended to be.

After that first moment, during our sleepless night on the futon, I felt this sensation often. I tried to explain it to John, but I didn't really know how to articulate it, and he didn't know what I was talking about. Then, of course, came the car accident, and after that I didn't need to explain.

We were headed north at the time, into the gorgeous deciduous forests of upper New England. The trees in that part of the country put on a truly awesome autumn display. The sky is so blue it makes you want to cry, and the leaves look like they're on fire. The traffic out of Boston and into the backwoods of New Hampshire is pretty much bumper to bumper, although it moves along at a good, fast clip. Everyone goes north in the autumn. The volume and brilliance of the foliage is a major topic of conversation at the innumerable wine and cheese parties that kick off every academic year. John and I didn't own a car, but we were tired of being left out of these discussions, so we'd rented one to go up to New Hampshire. We were planning to spend a few days at a cabin with some friends, to celebrate surviving registration and returning to our native time zone.

We had left Massachussetts behind us and were cruising along on the freeway to Franconia when, for no apparent reason, a battered Chevy truck pulled off the shoulder, at right angles to the flow of traffic, and stopped directly in our path. There was no room, no time, to do anything. I heard John give a strangled yell as our car yawed violently and began to spin like a top across our lane and into the path of the oncoming traffic. The Chevy loomed up at me through the passenger window, then disappeared into a blur of leaves, which disappeared behind an eighteen-wheeler, then leaves again, then a Volkswagen bus, leaves, cars, leaves, cars, leaves. On our way home, we would stop at the site and see from the skid marks that we had spun around at least four times, careening across both lanes of the busy highway twice. I still can't see any way we could have done that without being hit, probably several times. But we did.

The odd thing is that I never had any doubt we were completely safe. I remember being mildly concerned that the spinning motion might make Katie carsick. I tried to turn around to look at her, strapped into her car seat behind me, but I was pinned against my own seat by a centrifugal force stronger than anything I had ever felt. I couldn't even move my head. So I just relaxed and watched the leaves go by.

All of this took about two seconds, maybe three. As we Tilt-A-Whirled back into our own lane and onto the shoulder, I could hear the brakes screaming and feel the car slowing down. Then there was a loud *pop!* and we were all thrown forward against our seat belts. We had hit the wooden post of a stop sign, breaking it in two and denting our bumper. I watched the top half of the sign tremble, sway, and collapse into the dust like a martyred lollipop.

We sat in silence for a minute, taking a mental inventory of our limbs and digits, before John reached forward to turn off the ignition. His hands, like his face, had gone bone white. I felt fine, except that my seat belt had clamped down too tight. I also detected a strange sensation in my lower abdomen, as though someone was pressing a firm but gentle thumb against my bladder. I seemed to remember having felt it before, but I couldn't remember when. I looked over at John. He was clutching the steering wheel as though his life depended on it, which, come to think of it, it did.

"I lost control!" he gasped, as though this were an unfathomable mystery.

"Uh-huh," I said. I turned around and looked at Katie, who was beaming at me from her car seat.

"Whee!" she said.

I laughed. "That was fun, wasn't it, Boofus?"

"Do again?" she asked hopefully.

"No, honey, I'm not sure Daddy *could* do it again." I turned to smile at John, because the whole situation seemed so interesting. My reaction could have come from shock, I suppose, but all I remember is an entirely inappropriate—though rock solid—sense of well-being. John was still staring straight ahead, gripping the wheel.

"I lost control," he repeated. He was trembling.

I began to wonder why John was making such a big deal about this. True, it was probably the first time since he was potty trained that John had ever lost control of anything. But it was utterly obvious to me that we had never been in any danger. The Bunraku puppeteers wouldn't have allowed it. At this thought, the hair began to prickle all over my body, because I could feel them again. They were all around us, all around the car, as powerful and invisible as an ocean current. And I suddenly knew why John was so thoroughly spooked. He hadn't lost control to the forces of nature. He had lost control to *them*.

There was a sudden, loud rap on the window by my head. John and I jumped so violently that only our seat belts saved us—again—from bashing our heads against the windshield. I turned to see two old men in overalls standing by the car, peering into the interior. I rolled down my window.

"The grace a God was with you then!" one of the men told us in a thin, accusatory voice, as though we had stayed out too late after the prom.

"The grace a God," echoed the other man. He was wearing a fluorescent orange hunting cap, and his voice was thick and slow. He had the strangest pale-silver eyes I had ever seen. I could tell immediately that he was not, shall we say, fully cooked.

"Car still runnin'?" asked the first man.

John turned toward him and gave him a huge smile. The more upset John is, the happier he acts. It's a Harvard thing.

"Everything's great!" he said, grinning like a maniac. He turned the key, and the car vroomed obediently.

"Everything's great!" the man in the hat repeated in a singsong voice. I couldn't stop looking at him. Retarded people had always filled me with revulsion. I wanted to look away, but I couldn't. The puppeteers wouldn't let me.

"Okay!" John chirped, like Rebecca of Sunnybrook Farm on an especially magical day. "I guess we'd better get going!" He put the car in reverse and backed slowly, cautiously, away from the stump of the stop sign.

The first man grunted, turned, and walked away from the car. The one in the hat was still watching me.

"He's a good baby, ma'am," he said. "You take good care of that baby."

I remember being puzzled that he had taken Katie for a boy. I thought of correcting him but decided it wasn't worth the effort. For some reason (probably the aftereffects of the accident), I felt gooseflesh rising on the back of my neck. I gave the man an artificial smile, mostly because I was so glad we were getting away from him. The pressure against my bladder seemed to grow stronger, and I suddenly remembered when I had felt it before. It was the first sign I'd had that I was pregnant with Katie.

John was driving very carefully, searching the road intently. "Did you see that idiot?" he said.

"The guy in the hat?" I said.

John glanced at me as though I were short a few brain cells myself. "No," he said. "The guy in the *truck*."

"Oh, the truck. Yeah, sure . . ."

"He pulled right into my lane!" John fumed. "*Right into* it!"

"I know, honey," I said, trying to sound soothing. "It was all his fault."

"I ought to report him," said John. He wasn't trembling anymore, but his shirt was soaked with sweat. I thought about continuing to play the supportive wife, encouraging him to vent his testosterone rage on the enemy trucker, but I was too preoccupied searching my memory for any acts of indiscretion involving birth control.

"Let it go, John," I said. "He's long gone."

We'd been very careful, I was sure we had. I was particularly cautious about contraception since my physiology had proven incompatible with birth control pills. That night in the apartment, when the ocean current had caught me and carried me along with it, John and I had been as conscientious as usual. But I was well aware that the methods of contraception at my disposal were not fail-safe.

"He's going to kill somebody," John brooded. A car passed us on the left, and he jerked the steering wheel much too hard to the right.

"Just relax," I said. "It was a freak accident." I was trying to make my voice sound the way Mister Rogers's does when he's telling viewers they can't go down the drain, but it cracked with tension. John didn't notice. He was too busy slamming on the brakes to avoid a falling leaf.

We went along that way for the next fifty miles, John driving like someone's grandmother, while I did my best to reassure him that everything was fine. But deep down in my heart—well, all right, deep down in my bladder—I knew better.

3

∾ Adam deals with many things more graciously than I do. Take illness, for example. My first clue that he isn't feeling well is usually a polite knock on my bedroom door in the middle of the night. After a pause, just as I'm telling myself that I didn't hear anything and should go back to sleep, a small, gruff voice will rasp, "Mom, U'm gick."

I'll drag myself awake to find him standing by my bed, fraught with some horrific assortment of symptoms: blazing fevers, rashes that turn his usually flat little face into a topographical map of Nepal, chest coughs that sound like gang warfare between two prides of lions. Adam's immune system is weaker than a normal nine-year-old's, and every germ he catches rollicks gaily through his body, holding orgies of self-reproduction and sending enthusiastic invitations to others of its kind. When Adam gets gick, he gets really, really gick.

Gick, if you haven't figured it out by now, is Adam's word for *sick.* He has learned to speak fairly well in the last few years, but the muscles of his mouth aren't formed for our language, so he often uses his own. Adamic, we call it. It is a strange dialect, in which syllables are often reversed or replaced with random consonants, sound effects, and gestures. Our youngest daughter, Elizabeth, who learned it along with English, understands Adamic quite well, and often acts as my interpreter. But I don't need a translation when my son wakes me up in the night. "Gick," he'll repeat patiently. There isn't a trace of a whine in his voice, just a touch of regret. He is clearly sorry to have disturbed me.

Eventually I get out of bed, and we go down the hall together, Adam holding my hand in his small, dry, stubby fingers. We stand in the doorway of his bedroom and assess the damage. This is what always amazes me: if he's thrown up, he will have done his best to clean the room before involving me. "Bleah," he will explain, flipping his hand from his mouth outward, as though the smell alone weren't enough to tell me what happened. "I keen."

"Yes," I'll say. "You cleaned up. Thanks, buddy. Good boy."

Then Adam, ill and weary as he is, helps me spray the rug with cleanser, scrub out the stain, and change his sheets. He gamely swallows a dose of Tylenol, says "Unkoo, Mom," and flops down on his pillow, already asleep. The genetic weakness of his muscles (hypotonia, the doctors call it) lets his body fall into strange shapes, as though he has been dropped out of a plane to his death; legs twisted under him, undersize head bent too far back, chunky little arms flung wide. His small, slanted eyes flicker behind their lids as he begins to dream. Watching him, I think he is the most beautiful child I have ever known.

The point here is this: Adam's gentlemanly stoicism in the face of illness did not come from me. My method is to rage against the dying of the light, and I believe in getting started as soon as the light displays the tiniest flicker. When I was Adam's age, I would howl and whimper in protest through the duration of the most minor illness. I think I believed that if I could only make the adults as miserable as I was, they would arrange to give me general anesthesia. Perhaps my reaction to pregnancy was Nature's way of avenging my parents for the trauma they experienced during my childhood.

Now, I am not generally a bitter person. I don't even have to try to rejoice in the good fortune of others. Usually. But every time I hear a woman say something like "Oh, golly, for the first four months I didn't even know I was pregnant," I find my hands clenching into fists and my upper lip curling back to display my teeth—which, by the way, had to be substantially reconstructed after each of my three pregnancies because the enamel had dissolved under a constant barrage of stomach acid. It never took me four months to figure out I was expecting. Oh, no indeed. From the moment Mr. Sperm and Ms. Egg first encountered each other in my fallopian tubes—before they even had time to make any informed decision about going *steady,* let alone forming a biological unit—I could sense them conspiring to make my life a hell on earth.

The nausea was the worst part. Saying that I was nauseated during pregnancy is like saying that Hurricane Andrew was "breezy with scattered showers." This was not the morning queasiness my many pregnancy books told me to expect. It wasn't even the pretty awful feeling you get when you contract an intestinal virus. I am talking about an epic nausea, a vast and overwhelming nausea, a nausea that, in my humble opinion, deserves to be chronicled in song and legend for centuries to come. Seven years after my last day of pregnancy, I still have to swallow hard just writing about it.

Unfortunately, things did not stop at the digestive level. Pregnancy seemed to attack every system and organ in my body. A week or so after Katie was conceived, I took what I thought was a bold step forward and was stunned to see my foot swing out about five inches and plop, like a well-boiled noodle, back to the ground. I had always been very active, had run a few honest-to-goodness marathons in my time, and was used to pushing through pain and fatigue. But when my body was in its reproductive mode, nothing else worked. It was that simple. Throughout each pregnancy, I went around with my teeth clenched, trying to behave like a Harvard woman—firm, strong, dauntless, intimidating—but looking and moving like Deng Xiaoping just before they fired up the cremation furnace.

Then, of course, there was the issue of fainting. I go hot with shame whenever I remember the many times and places my pregnant self passed out. There was never much warning: I would be puttering along pretty well, then suddenly everything would go an unpleasant shade of green and I would pitch over like a bowling pin, to wake up several seconds later on yet another inappropriate horizontal surface.

On most of these occasions, the people around me assumed that I was simply having a normal reaction to the final stages of a tragic drug addiction, and paid no attention. A few thought to call the police, but most exercised that iron-willed inattention that is so basic to the culture of the northeastern seaboard. I remember, for example, that when I fainted in a hardware store, several customers had to step over me to find the right hammer. I was intensely relieved that they pretended not to notice me. Other than these small mercies, I can't say that I found much to celebrate in my physical experience of gestation.

Years after my final pregnancy "cleared" (I borrow this term from the personnel at the Harvard University Medical Clinic), I was diagnosed with an autoimmune disease that explains the severity of my "morning sickness." By then we had moved away from Boston, first to our hometown in Utah, where I wrote my doctoral dissertation, then to Arizona. We chose Arizona simply because it was warm and beautiful (reasons that would not have impressed us at all before Adam came along), and we set up our lives to be as stress-free and comfortable as possible. By the time my medical condition was diagnosed, these changes had already made the symptoms much easier to manage.

But back in 1987, when John and I took our trip to New Hampshire, my life was not arranged to accommodate ill health. I had no idea that there was a name, let alone any treatment, for the condition that made my body go wildly haywire during pregnancy. I wasn't even thinking about it. As we drove our dented, rented car away from the scene of the accident, I quite deliberately refused to admit that the peculiar feeling in my abdomen was accompanied by an overall sense of the Deng Xiaoping weakness I remembered from the months I was pregnant with Katie.

We eventually made it, bashed-up car and all, to the cabin we had rented. The northern New Hampshire woods were beautiful, in that impossibly rich, fecund way that New England forests are beautiful. The air was full of the smells of pine and loam and autumn leaves, a combination that ordinarily would have sent me reeling with delight. The first morning we were there I went out for a walk, and did in fact do a little reeling. The delight part, however, was conspicuously absent. I felt woozy and ill but told myself it was only a little flu bug, possibly something I'd picked up in Japan.

The second day, I was sitting on the cabin steps watching Katie play in the leaves when John rushed up to report that there was a moose, an actual live wild moose, standing in a streambed not a hundred yards from us. Well, this stirred my nature-loving blood, I can tell you. I leapt off the steps and ran to see the moose, ducking swiftly and noiselessly through brush and brambles like the Last of the Mohicans. At least I meant to. What I actually did was waddle forward a few steps like a penguin and collapse.

John, who had already pivoted to lead the moose-watching brigade, stopped dead and looked at me uncertainly. I looked at John uncertainly. Katie looked at us both uncertainly.

"Oops," I said, grinning at them, my Fang personality taking over to put all our minds at rest. I yanked myself to my feet with a burst of willpower and added, "I think I need to get something in town."

And so, after watching the moose through binoculars for a while, we all piled in the car and headed to a nearby village. We found a small pharmacy, and John stayed in the car with Katie while I went in to look for a home pregnancy test. Not that I actually thought I might be pregnant, you understand. There was no way I could be pregnant. I found myself arguing with some faceless audience in my mind—the Bunraku puppeteers, I suppose—insisting that, with all the precautions I had taken, I was more likely to be attacked by killer bees than to get pregnant. I just wanted to rule out the possibility, to get rid of the uneasy feeling that had been nagging me since the car accident.

I bought a test and went back to the car. John didn't ask what was in the little pharmacy bag; I had simply told him that I wasn't feeling well and needed some over-the-counter medication. We drove back to the cabin, where some of our dearest friends from undergraduate days had arrived in our absence. I scurried into a back bedroom and yanked the pregnancy test out of its wrapper, intending to put my mind at rest then and there. Of course I couldn't. Such tests require a urine sample from the day's first piddle, or as my particular test put it, "your first morning stream." While I appreciated the poetic nature of this instruction (it made me think of dawn light on rushing waterfalls and crystal mountain brooks emanating from my very own bladder), it was extremely frustrating. When I'm not feeling tip-top, my small stores of patience tend to dry up altogether.

I slept restlessly that night, thinking about the intense semester that would begin the day we returned to Cambridge and worrying about the unpleasant dizziness I felt even when I was lying down. At 6:00 A.M., after staring at the ceiling for a couple of hours, I got up and took the pregnancy test into the bathroom. I produced an entirely unromantic First Morning Stream, mixed it with the chemicals that had come in the little plastic test tube, and waited. It was supposed to take five minutes. If the liquid remained clear, I was not pregnant. If it turned blue, I was.

I checked my watch, then looked deliberately out the small window at the lovely autumn foliage. I decided to give the test ten minutes, instead of five, before definitely concluding I was not pregnant—I had always been conscientious and wanted to be absolutely sure I allowed sufficient time. I didn't even think about what I would do if the test came back positive. There was always the unarticulated but clear possibility of a quick, early abortion—but, of course, I wouldn't need that. I looked at my watch again. Thirty seconds. I yawned, stretched—and froze. Out on the very edge of my peripheral vision was a flash of blue. I turned slowly toward the test tube, and there it stood, a tiny, crystalline column of turquoise liquid, blushing slowly into a deep royal blue.

It was at that moment that the feeling came. Before I had a single thought, before I was even able to process the meaning of the blue vial, it flowed clear through my body like warm honey, taking my breath away. And instead of thinking through my Plan for Life and clearing out time for the abortion, I found myself lost in a memory so vivid it seemed I had moved back in time.

During my freshman year at Harvard, I ran for hours every day. I would set out for a run—six miles, ten miles, twenty—in howling blizzards, in the middle of the night, sometimes with my backpack full of books still strapped to my shoulders. I ran because I needed to; it muted my anxieties and eased my loneliness. Running was the only thing I did that year that wasn't completely dominated by fear, or perhaps it was the only time I responded to my omnipresent fears in a way that felt like escape. I ran no matter what the weather, and the winter was terrible. There were times when the wind would blow me backwards or sideways in midstride. There were days when the tips of my toes froze black and I had to wrap pieces of plastic bags around my hands so that my fingers wouldn't do the same.

In March, as the temperature rose above freezing and the sun began to linger beyond midafternoon for the first time in months, running became an intoxicating pleasure. A Boston Marathoner told me that you could tell it was springtime in New England because the saps were beginning to run. He was right. The warmer weather brought hordes of joggers into my usual path along the Charles River, and I began to look for less crowded routes. That is why, one Sunday in early April, I found myself in the Boston Common, a wide, grassy park in the middle of the city. I had already run across Cambridge, over the long bridge by MIT, and through the seedy Boston neighborhoods near Chinatown. The city was unusually empty that morning, very still in the warm dawn light.

I reached the Common at about 8:00 A.M., and as I jogged onto the path beneath the yellow-green leaves of budding trees, I began to notice strange things. There were people in the park, but not the usual gangs of spiky-haired teenagers and scruffy, homeless beggars. The people were in groups, all elaborately clothed; the men and boys in suits, the women and girls in dresses the color of flowers. There was a kind of quiet decorum to the whole scene that was quite unlike anything I had seen in Boston. A woman in a lavender gown went past me, pushing a stroller. Tied to the stroller handle was one end of a braided leash. At the other end walked a small dog in a checkered vest and a tie. As they went by I saw that the stroller contained not a baby but a large gray rabbit wearing a straw bonnet. I stopped dead in my tracks—something I never did during a run—and stared.

It was then that the sound began. I felt it before I heard it. The soft ground seemed to swell like something breathing, and through the soles of my feet, up my legs, and into my body rose a thrumming vibration that seemed to bond me with the earth. The exquisite sensation grew more and more intense for several seconds before I began to hear it. It was the clearest, purest tone I had ever heard. As it rose in pitch, I finally realized that it was the sound of a bell.

Boston's bell makers (like Paul Revere) were famous for good reason. I have heard many bells in my time, but the best of them sound like bashing cooking pots next to the bells I heard that morning. The first one, the deep and almost inaudible one, was joined within minutes by dozens of others, but I never heard anything that sounded like a clapper striking metal. Nor did the sounds seem to come from any particular direction. Instead, the air simply filled with sustained, meltingly sweet tones, like angels singing. The whole scene was so strange and beautiful that tears began to run down my cheeks, faster than I could stop them. I stood in the Common surrounded by this glorious sound, watching the strange loveliness of beribboned people and animals, and seriously debated whether or not I had been transported to some bizarre but benevolent alternate universe.

By the time I got back to my dorm and realized that it was Easter Sunday, the impression had already been made. Despite the perfectly rational, ordinary reasons for that moment in the Boston Common, I had stored it in my memory as a glimpse into a magical world, and that image would never quite go away. It did, however, fade quickly into the realm of quirky and unusual experiences that I was sure had nothing to do with my Plan for Life. As the years went by, I sometimes found myself longing for that moment when I surrendered my common sense to enchantment, but I was far too logical to allow myself to go back there—until that morning in the New Hampshire woods, when I glanced at a tube of blue liquid and felt the magic flooding through me all over again.

By the time the five minutes had elapsed and the pregnancy test results were undeniably positive, I knew that I would not be scheduling an abortion. That was all I knew. I wasn't sure why I had made the decision to continue the pregnancy. I could feel the puppeteers around me, sounding their invisible bells in some inexplicable but irresistible celebration, and I strongly suspected that this meant I was losing my mind. I checked to see if I was still pro-choice. I was. I examined my internalized schedule for the upcoming year: my teaching, caring for Katie, intense classwork, John's travel. This was simply not the time for a baby, I thought. But at the word *baby,* the joyous carol swelled again, and the magic filled my eyes with tears. I stood up, teetered a little, and went to tell John that he was going to become a father for the second time.

4

If you ever need some heavy winter clothes at a good price, you should stop by the factory outlets in southern New Hampshire, on the road between Franconia and Boston. I still have some of the sweaters I bought there in 1987, right after I found out I was expecting Adam. They're good quality—pure wool and all that—and they were dirt cheap, especially considering how large they are. They aren't what I would choose for my usual wardrobe, but they were perfect at that time, when my objective was not style but camouflage. I intended to hide my delicate condition from all the folks at Harvard for as long as ever I could, and this meant swathing myself in so many yards of fabric that no one could tell whether I was shaped like Ichabod Crane or Luciano Pavarotti.

The factory-outlet shopping spree was John's idea. When I showed him the results of the pregnancy test, he reacted with a very long silence, followed by a shaky smile. Then he launched into an enthusiastic diatribe about how this was actually a pretty good time to have another baby. After all, he reminded me, we had always wanted two children. Graduate school gave us more flexibility than our future careers probably would. Furthermore, the baby would actually be born right at the beginning of the summer break, which meant that we would have three months to raise it from a plasma pet, then get it into day care before school started again. John babbled on like this for half an hour, his voice so full of forced confidence I thought he might become completely manic and start ricocheting around the room. I sat on the bed in our rented cabin and tried to make myself believe he was right. Then I threw up.

I made it crystal clear to John that the pregnancy was to be kept secret. The thought of my classmates and teachers finding out about it made me throw up again every time it crossed my mind. Since my academic focus was the sociology of gender, most of the people I interacted with at Harvard were staunch feminists. I had always considered myself a staunch feminist, too, but it had been clear since the moment I began my degree program that I did not fully meet the requirements. John and I had married young, by Harvard standards, and my first year as a Ph.D. candidate had been dominated by the struggle to finish enormous amounts of academic work while getting Katie through early infancy. This had led to many humiliating experiences, like the time I absent-mindedly covered a statistics assignment with Muppet Babies stickers, or the day one of my famous professors uttered the key word *baby* during a lecture and my milk let down, soaking the front of my shirt.

The academic year of 1987–88 was going to be my time to redeem my reputation, to put all the mommy stuff behind me and prove that I could be single-mindedly devoted to scholarship. Instead, there I was— a day before the semester started—staring down the barrel of yet another baby. The curious elation I had felt since taking the pregnancy test did not go away, but it quickly became marbled with grim fantasies of the things people at Harvard would say about me when my condition became known. I could hear them in my mind, comparing me to a rabbit, a brood sow, a member of some primitive tribe that hadn't figured out the connection between sex and reproduction. My imagination broadcast these comments at high volume as I plodded through the New Hampshire factory outlets.

Meanwhile, John was also buying clothes that did not match his style. He was preparing to enter the workforce as a Management Consultant. For this, he needed suits. John had never worn suits by choice. He was wedged into them frequently as a child; even his earliest baby pictures show him in three-piecers with little bow ties, his hair parted and Brylcreemed, looking like a tiny CEO. John's conservative, churchgoing parents loved to see him dressed this way. Every time we visited them, at Christmas or during the summers, they would murmur politely horrified comments about his clothing, his haircut, the stubble on his chin. They were disappointed to realize that Harvard is not an executive's fashion Mecca. Actually, it is quite the opposite. I think there is an implicit understanding at the university that too much attention to one's clothing signals a contemptible lack of focus on the mind. The John I fell in love with wore the typical Harvard clothes his mother loathed: hiking boots, moth-bitten sweaters, and jeans so worn they fit like loose blue skin.

In the autumn of '87, it looked as though John's days of slovenly comfort had come to an end. While I was in one store, glumly paying for a cardigan the size of Peru, John was in another becoming a model from one of those business hotel ads in airplane magazines. He bought two Brooks Brothers suits (one gray, one blue), some conservative ties, several white Arrow shirts, suspenders, socks, and Italian shoes. Then, to top it all off, he got his hair cut.

I had always loved John's hair. It was soft, curly, and very blond, and like most of the other students I knew, he allowed it to grow unpruned for entire academic years. When he returned to his parents' house the summer after his freshman year, John's mother had almost fainted at the sight of all that honey-colored hair curling into his eyes and over his collar. To humor her, he cut it all off before he allowed himself to be seen by her friends and neighbors. He did the same thing every summer thereafter, and it always made me sad. When we met just outside the dressing room at the Brooks Brothers outlet, his hair was shorter than I had ever seen it. He looked plastically perfect, exactly like every other business consultant I had ever met.

"So," he said triumphantly, "what do you think?"

I began to cry.

John would have been hurt by this if he hadn't known that during pregnancy I could be moved to tears by televised golf. Still, he was crestfallen. I think he expected me to be as proud as his mother had been on the day she first Brylcreemed his hair.

"Not good?" he said anxiously, looking in the mirror.

Katie crowed at him from her stroller. They had picked out the suits together.

"Boofus thinks I look good," said John defensively.

"You do look good," I said, still weeping. "You just don't look like *you.*"

John shrugged resignedly. "Well, I don't feel much like me," he said.

"But I've got to do this. I mean, now, with the . . ." He gestured meaningfully toward my stomach. "I've got to make this work, Marth."

I managed to rein myself back to a moist snuffle.

John forced a smile and put his arms around me. His suit felt strange against my cheek, and I worried about crying on it. I could feel the tension in his chest, as though the burden of a second child had already settled on him.

"I should probably get another suit," he said in a distant voice, looking at the racks of sober-colored wool around us. "It looks like I'll be living in them from now on."

As I look back, there are a few things about this scene that strike me as deeply ironic. John and I felt so trapped by the pregnancy, trapped by the necessity of making a home—not just for a young couple, not even for a couple with a baby, but for a family, an entire *family*: mom, dad, and *the kids*. Somewhere in my subconscious mind I know I was worried that I'd have to start baking. John felt himself slipping into the role of the Company Man, enslaved to an employer by the needs of his dependents. Neither of us would have believed that the little clump of cells creating itself inside my belly would ultimately lead us to our present lifestyle, where we spend most of our time wandering around in T-shirts, shorts, and, on formal occasions, beach thongs.

Another irony about our suit-buying adventure is that the love of the "corporate look" in John's parents seems to have skipped a generation, missing John altogether but bursting forth, splendiferously, in Adam. When he was tiny I had nightmares about Adam growing up to wear "retard clothes." These had been worn by every disabled person at the American Fork Training School, where my junior high school choir had gone to sing Christmas carols. For me, the annual goodwill trek had been terrifying. The children at the training school (who were lumped together indiscriminately, regardless of the differences in their abilities, needs, and interests) were prone to strange outbursts, lapses of attention, sometimes even violence. They also sported outfits of mesmerizing ugliness. Double knit was very big at the training school, as were the colors mustard, beige, and puce. In combination. Add to this a random sample of broken fasteners, and the occasional football helmet worn backwards, and you begin to get the picture. This is how I thought Adam was genetically destined to dress, and when he was very small I swore a mighty oath to keep him in Oshkosh overalls and little Guess! jeans until he was strong enough to physically resist me. Little did I know.

One day when Adam was four, he disappeared in a department store. After a frantic search I located him in the section labeled "Men's Better Business Attire." He was trying to drag two pin-striped suits into the fitting room without getting all tangled up in the legs, which were a good deal longer than his entire body. Adam protested violently when I took the suits away from him, stretching himself yearningly toward the clothing racks. By this point I had learned that there were times to simply let go of the reins and see what he did next, so I took him to the "Children's Formal Wear" section and showed him that the store actually carried suits in his size.

He has never returned to casual wear. Every day before Adam heads off to third grade, he spends about an hour coordinating his look. Some days he goes for *Miami Vice*—a blazer over jeans and an expensive T-shirt—but generally he prefers a professional-looking dark suit, a white shirt, and a tie. He's been doing this since he started preschool. We have absolutely no idea why. For the past three years he has taken an extra suit along with him in his backpack for his friend Joey, who also has Down syndrome. They look like a couple of weird little executives dashing around the playground. No one understands what they say to each other, but I think they're doing what all management consultants do: coming up with marketing strategies, negotiating intellectual-property agreements, pouring sand in each other's hair when communication breaks down.

When John and I go out to meet the school bus at the end of the day, Adam gives us the same look we used to get from John's mother, the Oh-my-lord-is-that-what-you're-*wearing*? look. And that's when we remember to put on our thongs. It would probably embarrass him less if we dressed the way most middle-aged people do. But Adam the fashion slave has set us free. He has only himself to blame.

5

✎ Once we'd returned to Cambridge, I managed to stay in denial for about a week. The nausea and the weakness were still tolerable, as long as I ate something every ten minutes or so. I was determined to simply ignore my morning sickness throughout this second pregnancy.

Fortunately, there was much to distract me. I had signed up for coursework that fit well with my interests: a seminar on the sociology of gender, classes on research methods and economic development, Japanese language. I had also been hired as a teaching fellow for an undergraduate course on the society of the Caribbean region. This job was somewhat unnerving to me, since it turned out that just about everyone who took the class was actually *from* the Caribbean and I had never even been there on vacation. I had agreed to teach the class because I greatly admired its professor, a brilliant man with incredible breadth and depth of knowledge and a sense of poetry rare among sociologists.

During that first week of classes, I met with this professor and his other teaching fellows in the Harvard Faculty Club, a venerable building where geniuses go to eat lobster bisque and match minds. The place was redolent of pipe smoke and food smells, airborne ipecac for someone as chock full o' hormones as I was. Clamping my teeth to keep my stomach from taking off for the Caribbean all by itself, I focused on the discussion of my responsibilities. I would be expected to attend lectures on Monday and Wednesday mornings, teach a Friday "section" of about twenty students, and grade exams and papers for the same group. Once that was settled, the conversation at the table turned to pleasantries. The professor mentioned that a former student of his, someone we all knew, had recently married and was now expecting a baby.

Here's the big problem with denial: it leaks. When you're trying hard not to talk about something, trying hard not even to *think* about it, that very thing begins to creep into places it never belonged, to spurt out at the corners of everything you say or do. I have always been especially likely to blurt out the unmentionable, and pregnancy exaggerated this trait, as it did just about every embarrassing quality I possess. At the mention of the mother-to-be, I began to babble like a brook.

"She's *pregnant*?" I heard myself say. "Good lord, who *isn't* pregnant? Seems like everyone I *know* is pregnant! Damn!"

Everyone at the table looked at me, with a befuddled expression. I suddenly remembered the way I felt the first time I went skiing. I had expected to have trouble going fast, but I immediately learned that going fast on skis isn't the problem. The problem is stopping.

"I don't know what all these people think they're doing, getting pregnant all the time," I rattled on. "And those damn maternity clothes! Are they ugly enough? Have you seen those 'Baby on Board' T-shirts? They're ridiculous. And furthermore . . ." I managed to trail off into a grumble and finally brought myself to a grinding halt. The others at the table took a collective deep breath. *Whatever,* their faces said. *There are a lot of weird people around this place.* Appalled at my outburst, I excused myself and went to the rest room to throw up.

⌐ By the second week of the semester, it was already becoming difficult to lead a normal life. I could barely lift Katie; my arms felt as though they had been filled with Jell-O. I was consumed by an overpowering desire to sleep, but whenever I got a chance to lie down, the nausea made it hard to relax. One day I fainted on the lawn outside Memorial Hall, an elaborate architectural monstrosity built around the time of the Civil War. As I lay there in my very large clothes, watching the bright autumn leaves flutter through the air above me, I realized that looking like a stoned Annie Hall was not my biggest problem. There was only one week left until John's first trip to Asia. He would be gone for two full weeks. How in the world was I going to keep up with work and school while taking care of Katie?

The previous year John and I had managed to attend classes and still cover all our own child-care needs. We had scheduled our classes at different times so that we could pass Katie off like a relay baton as we alternated between home and campus. On a typical day, I would walk a mile to my first class while John gave Katie breakfast. Immediately after that class I would run home and buzz the intercom to let John know I had reached the lobby of our apartment building. By the time I arrived on the tenth floor, John would be waiting by the elevators with Katie in his arms. I would grab her, John would grab the elevator, and he would run to *his* first class of the day. When his class ended I would be waiting by the classroom door with Katie in a backpack. We'd switch the pack without even taking her out of it, and John would head home with her while I skittered into a nearby room for my next class. This went on all day, every day. We had been tired beyond belief that year—had to eat a large batch of chocolate chip cookies every single day, just to keep up our strength. There was no way I could match anything like this level of activity while I was pregnant.

John and I had also made a fatal planning mistake when he accepted the Asian consulting assignment. We had assumed that we would be able to hire a decent baby-sitter without any trouble. We hadn't had the money for this luxury before, but John's consulting would get us out of the starving-student income range, and this year we were ready to pay a good price for a reliable sitter. It never occurred to us that we might not be able to find someone like this—after all, we had both had college students as baby-sitters when we were children, and Cambridge is packed with college students. Unfortunately, we failed to consider the fact that the city where we grew up, while definitely a college town, is also 90 percent Mormon. Permit me to generalize: college students in Utah like to baby-sit, but college students in Massachusetts do not.

We got only one reply to the listings we placed in the many student newspapers and employment centers in our area. This candidate proved to be a deathly pale teenager who dressed completely in black, never made eye contact, and spoke only in a hushed monotone. It was obvious to me she was a heroin addict, probably with Mob connections, who was just waiting for John and me to depart so that she could sell our daughter to slave traders in Pakistan. Nevertheless, I was so desperate that

I actually left Katie with her a few times. Nothing went obviously wrong, although I still have a little money saved up for Katie's therapy in case she ever starts having flashbacks of that bizarre, black-clad young woman sacrificing pigeons on the window ledge of our apartment. In any case, after two days she stopped showing up, and when I tried to call her, I found that her phone had been disconnected. Thinking it all through as I lay on the grass outside Mem Hall, I decided that I had to find a good day-care center near the campus.

This turned out to be a lot like finding a piece of the True Cross. My friends and acquaintances had heard rumors that there were day-care centers around Harvard. Some claimed that they had heard tiny, high-pitched voices in certain buildings, and a couple of people swore they had actually seen such centers in operation, but no one had ever, say, been able to photograph one. After questioning several people, I finally called the information number for the Boston area and asked the operator to list every day-care center north of the Charles River.

To my delight, one of these centers operated out of an old student-soldier barracks Harvard had built just after World War II. The building was about a block from William James Hall, where most of my classes and my office were located. The next closest day-care center was three miles from campus. The rest were much more distant. This would have been fine—if John and I had owned a car. As I checked my list of addresses, I contemplated the prospect of dressing Katie in winter gear, pushing her stroller to the nearest taxi stand or subway entrance, commuting to a day-care center, commuting back, hiking from the subway entrance to the campus, all in time to show up for morning class. As laborious as it sounded, my nonpregnant self could have done it. But with me functioning like Popeye during the Great Spinach Famine, I knew it was impossible.

I called the one geographically feasible day-care center with my fingers crossed, hoping it wasn't run by a bevy of pasty, funereal, murmuring baby-haters. It wasn't. The woman who answered the phone sounded warm and competent, like Mary Poppins with a Boston accent. As for the day-care center, she described it as state of the art, a veritable Eden for a few lucky tots and their parents. There were only twelve children in each age-group (infants, toddlers, preschoolers), and there were no fewer than four teachers for each group. In addition, every child's parents had to do weekly duty as volunteer teachers, so that on any given day there was at least one adult for every two children. Mary Poppins hadn't even finished describing the operation before I sang out, "That's enough! Sign me up!"

She chuckled. "Well, I'm glad you feel that way. Could you give me your name and phone number?"

I gave them to her.

"All righty," she said. "And when are you expecting to have a child?"

I was stunned. I thought no one but John and I knew about my condition. Did I somehow *sound* pregnant?

"Um, well, it's due sometime in June, I guess," I stammered.

"Oh!" said Mary. "Then you're already pregnant!" Her voice was concerned.

"Yes," I said slowly, hating to admit it out loud. "I am."

"And the baby's due in June?"

"That's right." I still couldn't figure out why she was so interested in a fetus. I thought day-care centers concerned themselves primarily with children who'd gotten past that gills-and-a-tail stage of development.

"June," she said dubiously. "That's a bit tight. I assume you'll want to start the baby out in our newborn age-group?"

I was rubbing my forehead, trying to figure out where this conversation was going. From the next room came the sound of Katie's crib mobile rattling, which meant she was waking up from her nap.

"Uh, yes, I suppose so," I said.

"Okay. Well, I can't guarantee there will be a space available, but I'll put you on the waiting list."

"Thank you."

"Is there anything else?"

"Uh, yes," I said. "Yes, there is. I already have a little girl, and I was hoping I could enroll her in your center . . . um . . . relatively soon."

"Mmm," said Mary. "How soon?"

I shrugged and went for it. "Today?"

A hearty peal of laughter rang from the phone.

"Seriously," she said. "When?"

"I was serious," I mumbled, listening to the cheerful cooing sound coming from Katie's room.

"Oh!" said Mary. She was embarrassed, I could tell—embarrassed that she had embarrassed me. She coughed, said, "I'm sorry," and continued carefully. "You must understand that getting a child into the center is very competitive. The usual waiting time is three to five years."

"Three to five years?" I repeated. "Your waiting list is three to five *years*?"

"That's right."

"But you don't take kids older than four!"

"Yes, I know." Mary Poppins sounded a little testy.

"Well then how can . . ."

"Most couples put their names on the list before they are actually— I mean physically—expecting a baby," she explained. "Of course they can't control exactly when they'll conceive, but once they do, there's a chance that the baby will be an appropriate age by the time their name comes up."

I felt as though someone had dumped a load of gravel on me. I slumped down and rested my head on my desk, still holding the phone to my ear.

"Okay." I sighed. "Well, I guess that's good to know. Thanks anyway."

"So do you still want your name on the list?" Her tone was delicate.

"Sure, I guess."

Mary must have heard the defeat in my voice. "You never know," she said gently. "Some people get boosted up because of the quotas."

"Quotas?" I murmured. I had closed my eyes. Suddenly, my desk seemed to be the perfect place for a long siesta.

"Race, gender, institutional affiliation," Mary said. "We have quotas for all of that. We're an equal opportunity center."

"Ah," I said.

"So sometimes, children who fit the right profile can get in quite quickly."

"Really. And how quickly is that?"

"Oh." She thought for a minute. "Maybe two years. Not very often, but sometimes it's only about two years."

"Fabulous," I said. "We'll be on pins and needles."

She laughed sympathetically. "I wish we could be of more help."

"Thank you. I appreciate that."

We hung up. I left my head on my desk for a few more seconds. There was nothing to do but keep calling through the list of day-care centers, but I didn't know how I would manage to get my daughter to them, even if they actually accepted her before she was old enough to vote. I could hear Katie talking in her bedroom.

"I'm awake now!" she sang. She pronounced it "avake," as though she had a baby German accent.

"Hi, Boofus," I said as I opened Katie's bedroom door. She was standing in her crib, holding the bars in her chubby fingers, her fine blond hair fuzzed out around her head like a halo.

"I yub you," she said, beaming.

"I love you too, kiddo." I picked her up and put her on my hip. She weighed only twenty pounds, but I felt as though I were lifting Godzilla.

I took her into our bedroom, set her—okay, dropped her—on the bed, and turned on the TV to *Sesame Street*. Then I flopped down on the bed myself. There was a stack of about twenty books by my pillow. I had a lot of studying to do. I picked up a dense monograph on Caribbean politics, but I was too worried to concentrate.

"What are we gonna do, Boof?" I asked.

"Big Bird," she said, pointing.

"Mm-hmm," I said, wondering if it might be better, after all, to end my pregnancy early. But that thought brought with it a shock of terrible grief, almost a physical pain. And then there was that other sensation, the one I had felt off and on ever since Adam's conception. As I lay there, I felt it rise around me like the tide.

If you have ever held two strong magnets close to each other, you know a little of this feeling. You see nothing, you hear, smell, taste nothing; yet the energy, the pull and push of these inert-looking objects, is undeniable. It drags things around, rearranges them, puts them in its own strange order. It reaches through blank space to touch without touching, to move without moving. I was becoming more and more conscious of this sensation. It filled the air around me. At times it was almost unnoticeable, but at other times it seemed to crescendo. I was simultaneously fascinated and frightened by it.

The phone rang.

I crawled across the bed and answered it.

"Mrs. Beck?" said the voice on the phone.

"Uh-huh," I said listlessly

"Is your child a Harvard-affiliated, eighteen-month-old Caucasian girl?"

I took the receiver away from my ear and stared at it. "Who is this?"

"It's the center," she said.

"What center?"

"The day-care center. We just spoke."

"Oh!" I finally recognized the Mary Poppins voice.

"Is your child a Harvard-affiliated, eighteen-month-old Caucasian girl?"

It took me a minute to sort through these descriptors. "Yes," I said at last.

A little squeal emerged from the receiver. "This is so wild!" said Mary. "I hadn't been off the phone with you two minutes when a family called in to cancel. They're moving across town. They had an eighteen-month-old, Harvard-affiliated Caucasian girl. If you'd like their slot, I'll give it to you."

I blinked. "You will?"

"Uh-huh!" Mary Poppins sounded mighty cheerful. In fact, she sounded a little blissed out, as though she'd just taken several Valium.

"Are you serious?" I said. She didn't seem like a sadistic practical joker, but I could hardly believe what she was doing. I pictured the three-to five-year waiting list, the virginal couples signing up for nonexistent children, the parents waiting desperately for slots.

"So, do you want it?" Mary gurgled happily.

"But," I said, "I don't think—I mean—what about . . ." I have this nasty fair streak. It doesn't come up often, but the idea of cutting in at the very front of a five-year line managed to rouse it. I intended, even wanted, to tell Mary Poppins that there was no way I could take the day-care slot away from people who had been waiting so long. But the magnetic sensation, the pull of those puppeteers, was reaching such a pitch that it clouded my mind and voice.

"We'll take it," I said.

6

⮌ John's first trip to Asia was scheduled for the second week in October. To prepare for it, he was expected not only to master a huge amount of information about his new employer and the client company but also to do two weeks of Harvard work ahead of time, in compensation for the days he would miss. Of course he never said so, but I had a strong suspicion that John found this ever so slightly daunting. Perhaps it was the way he paced around the apartment, reading his way through immense stacks of documents and rubbing his hand back and forth across his newly shorn head, or the fact that every time I asked him how his work was going, he got that strange, distracted look you see on the faces of Olympic sprinters just before the Big Race. He would stare into the middle distance, shifting his weight from foot to foot, answering questions like "Where did you put Katie's bottle?" with a terse yes or no. He started to look a little hollow around the eyes.

I'd never met anyone who could work like John. He was the kind of student who would hand in a final term paper after two weeks of a class, in order to get feedback and rewrite the thing, often several times, before the end of the semester. He had completed his undergraduate degree in three years, carrying a double major, and was one of about fifty students to achieve the coveted status of summa cum laude, "highest honors." I managed to love and accept him despite all this. At his graduation, where he wore the prized red tassel of the summa graduate and got to climb up on the stage to personally shake the hand of the college president, John's mother leaned over and whispered to me, "John isn't really very intelligent. He's just a hard worker." John and I had just become engaged, and I was trying very hard to integrate into his family. By the time we'd all spent his graduation day together, it was abundantly clear that no slacking was tolerated among the Beck clan. It was my first tiny taste of the subtle social dynamics that made John labor like a field hand at everything he did.

In the autumn of 1987, he was working hard enough to satisfy his family's wildest dreams. Aside from the full-time consulting job, John was taking a couple of classes and acting as a teaching fellow for an undergraduate course. Much worse, he had the brooding, loathsome monster that is a Ph.D. dissertation sitting heavily on his mind at all times. John's dissertation was about the Japanese tradition of "lifetime employment." His co-workers at the consulting company loved to ask about it so that they could feign deathly slumber as soon as he began to describe his research. Even now, a decade later, when John runs into people from the company, they will immediately say, "So, John, remind us about your dissertation. We remember how fascinating it was, but we've forgotten the details." John will roll his eyes and begin the description, knowing perfectly well that the questioners will immediately drop their chins to their chests and begin to snore extravagantly. I tell John that he should refuse to play, but he feels that would be like refusing to play peekaboo with a baby. It makes them so happy.

At any rate, one of the reasons John accepted the task of international liaison man, with its requirement that he commute between Boston and Singapore, was that he could stop in Japan en route and pick up necessary information for the dissertation. This did add three or four days to the duration of each Asia trip, but we didn't expect that to be a problem. At least, John didn't. By the time his first departure date arrived, I was getting worried. I worried every time I threw up, and every time I worried, I threw up again.

I plied this new hobby so often I'd long since run through a thesaurus of synonyms to describe it. My personal favorite was the term *ovorp* (pronounced "ov-vórp") which John had coined by spelling the name of our hometown backwards. I finally learned to ignore my occasional eruptions while having conversations with him, as though I had nothing worse than a serious burping problem: "So, what airline are you—excuse me (ovorp)—so what airline did you say you were flying?"

The morning John left for his first trip to Asia was especially bad. The queasiness had me up and reeling at the first blush of dawn. John had never gone to bed; he figured that he might as well get used to Singaporean time, which was exactly twelve hours different from Boston's. He had packed one of his Brooks Brothers suits and was wearing the other one. He stuffed the book he'd been reading into his hanging bag and kissed me good-bye, the distracted-sprinter look taking his gaze somewhere behind my head.

"I've got to go now," he said gently.

"Sure," I said.

"Well, *au revoir*." He smiled, nervously.

"*Bon voyage*," I said. French, the language of romance.

There was a long silence. Then John said, "Honey, are you going to let go of my arm?"

"Oh." I looked down at my hand, which was clutching the sleeve of his coat in a death grip. I peeled my fingers away.

"You'll be fine," he said, with that enormous smile that means he's really, really worried.

"Oh, I know," I lied. We kissed one more time, and he left.

ᴄ The first week wasn't so bad. It wasn't good, but it wasn't so bad. Every day I forced down some crackers and Coca-Cola. I got up on time each morning, feeling the way Lazarus must have after he'd been dead four days, and managed to push Katie's stroller to that wonderful day-care center in time to get to my own classes. It was true that I occasionally tossed my cookies during class period, and that I ended up lying on the floor behind a partition during the lectures for the Caribbean Society course, but by damn, I was there.

By the end of the week, though, things began to unravel. Attending classes was hard enough, but that was only the tip of the iceberg. Each class required an enormous amount of preparation, studying, paper writing, and similar chores, all of which were suddenly beyond me. My brain seemed to have turned almost all its attention to procreation; my memory went several volts dimmer, and my analytical powers dipped below levels I had observed in lab rats. I had to study twice as hard as usual, just to cover the material. My work was further limited by the fact that Katie needed my constant attention when not at the day-care center. She had inherited John's ability to function on five hours of sleep a night. By the eighth day of John's absence, I hit my first Death Spiral.

Death Spiral is the label I use to describe what happened when I was too nauseated to eat and became steadily more nauseated because I wasn't eating. I was dehydrated and almost delirious from the constant losing of lunch, and my body desperately needed food and fluid to calm itself. When this had happened during my first pregnancy, John had been there to rush to the rescue. He would hunt and forage in the small grocery store that occupied the first floor of our apartment building, looking for whatever peculiar assortment of foods I thought I could keep down. I never really experienced a craving for any food during pregnancy—I just wanted to stop eating forever—but there were certain items that sounded less unpleasant than others; odd things in odd combinations, like Spam and melba toast and kumquats. Once I'd eaten a food for a few days, it would inevitably become associated in my mind with nausea, and I would send John out to get something even more obscure.

After Katie was born, I looked back at this behavior with great embarrassment. How bourgeois to demand special delicacies, I thought, how . . . *stereotypical*. I vowed that if I ever got pregnant again, I would simply nibble on saltines and keep a stiff upper lip. This is the kind of decision that people make in badly written horror films, when they decide to go into the mausoleum or over to their unusual neighbors' house all by themselves. The entire audience is throwing popcorn at the screen, yelling, "Don't go! Stay home!" but on they march, straight into their own B-movie version of the Death Spiral.

It got me on Saturday. I had made it through Friday by the skin of my teeth, plopping over sideways every so often, dragging myself up with willpower and constant, internal reminders that I didn't have to go anywhere all weekend. I could rest. Friday night, Katie slept on the futon with me, partly because I was lonely and partly because I could no longer lift her into her crib. When I woke up in the morning, I was grateful to see her sitting up next to me with a half-full bottle, since this meant I could simply use the remote to switch on *Sesame Street,* and go back to sleep. When I woke up two hours later, I realized that it had been a mistake. My empty stomach was in the throes of such gut-wrenching nausea that I could hardly breathe. I tried to eat. No way. I couldn't swallow to save my life.

For the rest of that day I got steadily weaker and sicker. I managed to change Katie's diaper a few times, which is not something you really long to do when you're queasy. We sang some songs. We watched Mister Rogers. Katie acted bored and pent-up, but even at that age she was a very helpful person, and she could clearly tell I wasn't up to par. By evening I still hadn't been able to eat. I felt as though I were caught in a tidal wave of noxious hormones. When Katie fell asleep, an hour or so after sunset, I finally allowed myself to—very quietly—panic.

It never occurred to me to call anyone for help. First of all, I had long ago developed the habit of concealing all weakness from anyone around Harvard, and I never had the time to make friends away from the university. Then, too, I was determined to keep my pregnancy secret as long as possible. John was the only person in the world who knew how incapacitated I could get during pregnancy, and he was ten thousand miles away. As Katie slept beside me, I began to long for him, for his company, his strength, and his understanding.

I'm pretty sure that was the first time the Seeing Thing happened. That's what I called it—the Seeing Thing—although I'm sure there are more sophisticated words for it, defined in books I refuse to read because they're way too flaky. I was lying on the futon, staring up at the ceiling, biting the tip of one finger because I had found that pain distracted me from the morning sickness. The thought of the long night ahead, of the next morning, was terrifying. I was frightened for myself, but far more for Katie. She was already becoming a quiet, worried child, who watched me anxiously as I dragged myself around the apartment. My fear almost overcame me as I watched her sleep. I couldn't eat the food I could reach, couldn't get to any food I could eat, and didn't know what I would do if something didn't break the Death Spiral. I fought my emotions as long as I could and then, abruptly, lost control. Tears started running in two steady streams down my cheeks to my pillow. I began to miss John with an intensity that made me tremble—and then, suddenly, I was standing on a small, crowded street in Tokyo, watching the sun rise over a row of buildings.

I blinked, startled. It had been as instantaneous as a single frame of a movie shown in a dark theater, and much more vivid. I could feel the texture of the Japanese air against my face. The image had startled me right out of my doomsday mood, but only for a moment. I thought about it, decided it must be a memory, and went back to feeling deeply sorry for myself. I want John, I thought, like a child pining for its mommy. I want to be with John.

Poof.

The street ahead of me was crowded with the miniature trucks and immaculate taxis that always fill the streets of Tokyo. Ahead of me, five workmen in spotless blue uniforms and cotton leggings were clambering onto a fragile-looking bamboo scaffold, preparing to start their day's bricklaying. Steam and smoke rose in misty white billows from a *yaki tori* shop, where businessmen and "office ladies" were stopping to buy grilled chicken and soybean soup for breakfast. Then, suddenly, I was looking down another street, adjacent to the first. The rising sun burned splendidly before me. It shone through the silk of hundreds of brightly colored banners, making them glow like fluid stained glass as they fluttered in the light breeze.

I shook my head, and the image vanished. I looked around my bedroom, focusing very deliberately on the physical reality of the place. The shadows were still lengthening across the walls of our apartment. Katie still slept on the futon across from me, her small blond head cradled on one arm, her mouth slightly open. I still felt like the bottom of a toxic waste dump. But I had been somewhere else. I knew it—even though knowing it made me feel insane. I had been with John.

Once I had articulated this in my own mind, I set out to do some objective testing. If something is reliable, real, then it must be testable. That is the single thing that establishes the scientific validity of any hypothesis—if you create the same conditions, any number of times, you will get the same results. Being trained to think this way, I decided to repeat the experiment. I thought about how much I missed John. Nothing happened. I concentrated on my husband, repeating his name in my mind. I closed my eyes and tried to send my thoughts across the vast distance between us, imagined myself reaching across continent and ocean, waiting for the Seeing Thing to happen again. Nada. Zip. Zilch. I decided that the strange flash of Japanese scenery had been my imagination, ramped up by physical misery. Even so, I fell asleep wondering, buoyed slightly by the experience, as though I had taken a brief vacation.

🙠 I awoke to the ringing of the telephone. The room was light again, with the pale gray sunshine of dawn. When I reached for the phone, my head spun terribly. I had about as much arm strength as a chipmunk.

"Hello?"

"Hi, honey." John's voice came through the hissing wires of the transpacific phone lines. I felt a surge of relief that brought tears to my eyes again.

"Where are you?" I said, hoping irrationally that he was calling from the Boston airport.

"Tokyo," he said.

"Oh."

"How are you doing?" he said. It wasn't small talk; he was genuinely worried.

"Not well," I said stiffly.

"Are you okay?" His voice was anxious.

"No."

"Still sick?"

"Uh-huh." I was trying not to sound clingy, but it wasn't working at all. My eyes kept leaking all over the phone.

"You know," John said helpfully, "my mom says she was sick when she was pregnant, too, but if she just got herself up and kept moving, she'd stop noticing it."

I felt a rush of anger, mixed with shame. I had heard this repeatedly during my first pregnancy, from many women and a few obstetricians as well. I didn't know why all these people were so much tougher than I was, but I just didn't seem to have normal willpower.

"I'm sorry you feel so rotten," John said, after waiting a minute for me to respond. "I'll be back in just a couple of days, and I'll take care of you. Okay?" I could hear the restrained anxiety in his voice. He sounded very tired.

"It's okay," I said. "I'll be fine." I forced a little more energy into my voice. There wasn't anything he could do from that distance anyway. "So what have you been up to?"

I could almost hear him smile. "Well, I got a lot of research done here," he said.

"Did Singapore go well?"

"Oh, sure. They put me in a disgusting hotel, but work was fine."

"Good."

"I wish you'd been here this morning," he said, his voice taking on the kind of excitement it always did when he had seen something interesting. "I took a walk through Akasaka."

Akasaka is a district of Tokyo. John and I had often gone for walks there, with Katie in her backpack, while we were living in the city.

"There must have been some kind of festival," John went on, "because some of the streets were full of banners. I was there just when the sun was rising, and the banners—it almost looked like they were *glowing*, like they were made from neon or something."

I stared at the phone, feeling a slight prickling sensation across my scalp. "Did you see some workmen climbing a scaffold?" I asked.

John paused. "Well, uh, yeah," he said, sounding confused. "Why?"

The prickles tiptoed down my spine. "Was there a *yaki tori* stand?"

"Well, there might have been," he said. "Marth, are you all right?"

"I'm fine," I said. "I . . . uh . . . I think I've been there before." I briefly considered telling him about the Seeing Thing, but I was afraid he would think I was an idiot. John was as resistant as I was to the idea of anything paranormal. Growing up among religious fanatics in Utah had made us both wary.

"It was beautiful." John had returned to his story. "But I wish you and Boofus had been here. It's not the same when there's no one to share it with. I miss you."

"Me too," I said, wondering if the Seeing Thing would happen again right then. It didn't.

"Well, this is costing a fortune," said John.

"I know. I'll let you go."

"I love you," he said.

"I love you too," I told him. "Be safe."

We hung up. I felt like a deep-sea diver whose air hose had been severed. John wouldn't be home for two days. Katie stirred in her sleep, and her eyelashes fluttered. She would be awake soon, needing food, attention, a clean diaper. I wasn't sure I could manage it.

I decided to head for the kitchen immediately, to retrieve some food, so that Katie wouldn't have to watch me trying to run this little errand. I tried to stand up, but I had no equilibrium left, and I pitched over onto the floor. I crawled to the doorway and used the frame to pull myself up. Then I set one shoulder against the wall, leaning heavily, and scraped my way to the kitchen.

I knew I had to eat. The Death Spiral would only get worse until I did. I reached the kitchen, opened the refrigerator, and immediately vomited into the sink. Of course, my stomach was empty, so there wasn't much of a mess to clean up. I filled one of Katie's bottles with milk and found a package of animal crackers she could munch on. There was nothing I thought I could hold down. I hadn't been able to absorb food or liquid for almost forty-eight hours. I knew that prolonged dehydration could affect the fetus I was carrying. I began to think seriously about calling an ambulance, but it seemed so idiotic. We had the grocery store, Food Shak, just an elevator ride away. I considered it for a moment, wishing intensely that I could go there without actually having to put clothes on my body and stand up in the elevator.

Poof.

I was in the entryway to Food Shak, studying the overcrowded shelves, glancing over at the wizened little man who ran the cash register. Most of the packages on the shelves made my stomach lurch, but there were a few things—a bottle of raspberry juice, a package of rice cakes, a small cube of cheddar cheese—that didn't look so bad.

I slumped over the sink counter, head spinning, feeling loonier than ever. Naturally, I could picture the grocery store. I had been there hundreds of times. But the image had been so real, so *present*. I dry-heaved into the sink a few more times, shaking my head at my own delusions.

The kitchen of our small apartment was right next to the hallway door. As I puttered out of the kitchen, I heard a brisk knock. I groaned. It had to be the manager, or maybe the elderly lady who lived down the hall. The outside door of our apartment building was always locked; visitors had to buzz the intercom and identify themselves before someone in the apartment could release the lock and let them in. No one had buzzed our intercom. I shuffled over to the door with great reluctance. I didn't want to talk to the manager, and I certainly wouldn't be running any errands for the neighbor lady, though I had done so many times before. I looked through the peephole and frowned. All I could see was a mass of brilliantly red, curly hair. I opened the door, wondering if someone had the wrong apartment.

"Hi, Martha!"

The woman standing in the hallway was familiar to me, though not very. I had to search my pregnancy-dimmed memory for her name. Sibyl, I thought at last. Sibyl Johnston. Her husband, Charles Inouye, was a graduate student in the East Asian Studies Department. Their first child had been born at about the same time as Katie. Sibyl and I had met at a party when both of us were vast with child, and had spent the evening talking about morning sickness and laughing so hard at each other's jokes that I was afraid we'd both go into labor. That was all I knew about Sibyl, except that I was terribly embarrassed to be standing in front of her wearing little but an unwashed bathrobe.

Sibyl didn't seem even slightly perturbed. She grinned, her red hair bouncing around her face, and held out two large grocery bags from Food Shak.

"I was just passing by," she said, "and I got thinking about all the stuff we ate while we were pregnant, and I decided I'd get you some."

I squinted at her. This was not normal acquaintance behavior, particularly not in the emotionally distant culture of New England.

"Look," said Sibyl, peering into the grocery bags. "I got you some raspberry juice, and some rice cakes, and some cheese . . ." She laughed suddenly, her fair skin going pink. "I don't know why, I just thought I'd do it. Am I way out of line here?"

I still hadn't said a word. I was slumped against the wall, my mouth hanging open, the prickles crawling across my scalp and down my spine. And then, to my horror, I realized that tears had formed in my eyes again, and were spilling out onto my cheeks.

"Are you all right?" She was looking at me with concern.

"Thank you," I managed to gasp. I was not used to accepting help, and still less used to letting anyone see me cry. But even my tremendous funds of self-importance were beginning to give way. "I . . . uh . . . I really needed . . ." I couldn't control the tears any longer. I put my hands over my face and sobbed.

Sibyl Johnston, the relative stranger, took a step into my apartment, set one of the grocery bags on the floor, and put a strong arm around my shoulders just as I was about to pass out. "You okay?" she asked.

"I'm pregnant . . . again . . . can't eat," I gasped.

"All right, then." Sibyl has a low, strong voice, the kind of voice that could calm a crowd in the middle of a terrorist attack. "Let's feed you," she said. She propped me against the wall cautiously, as though I were a rag doll she was setting aside for a moment, and bustled into my kitchen with the two bags of food.

I stood there dazed, half-thinking about the Seeing Thing, half afraid to think about it. Once again, I was consumed by the eerie impression that my life was completely under control—but not *my* control. I watched Sibyl, who was quickly unloading every type of food I had just selected during my brief, incorporeal visit to Food Shak, and wept as much with bewilderment as with relief.

7

Sibyl stayed with me for over an hour, playing with Katie, bathing her, and changing her diapers, while I gradually relaxed enough to sip some raspberry juice. She did all of this in a pragmatic, unsentimental way, as though she had been planning it for weeks, as though it were the most ordinary thing in the world. Sibyl's matter-of-fact demeanor was the only thing that kept me from being utterly overwhelmed by her kindness. But Sibyl was far from finished. I found that out the next morning, when a buzz from the intercom woke me up.

I got out of bed carefully, still feeling queasy and weak, but not nearly as bad as I had the day before. The grip of the Death Spiral had been broken. I walked gingerly to the intercom and pressed the talk button.

"Hello," I said. "Who is it?"

"Hi, Martha. It's me again." Sibyl's voice came through, somewhat obscured by static. "And I've got Deirdre with me—Deirdre Hennesy."

I thought I remembered being introduced to the woman I'll call Deirdre Hennesy at the same party where Sibyl and I had met. I winced. This was not the morning I would have chosen to strike up a new acquaintance. I looked like road kill.

"Um . . . I'm not really dressed," I stammered into the intercom.

The answer came from a new voice, higher than Sibyl's. "Martha, it's Deirdre. Listen, don't worry. I'm pregnant too, and I look like hell."

"She really does," Sibyl confirmed.

"Well, thanks a million," said the other voice.

There seemed to be no polite option but to invite them up.

It took Sibyl and Deirdre about a minute to ride the elevator up ten stories. That was just enough time for me to brush my grimy hair and look despairingly around at the mess in my apartment. Books and papers were stacked on every horizontal surface. Katie's toys were scattered on the floor. Dust mice had formed in all the corners—large ones, more like dust German shepherds. I knew Sibyl would be understanding, but I hated the fact that there was anything about me that demanded her understanding, anything imperfect or disreputable. As for Deirdre, I seemed to remember that she was sort of a Martha Stewart type, very beautiful and aesthetic. There was no time to make myself or my home look presentable.

"Hiya!" Sibyl grinned at me as I let them in. "We're here for breakfast." As before, she was carrying a large bag full of food. I began to wonder if she just walked around that way, like Johnny Appleseed, looking for hungry pregnant women.

"We're going Continental today," said Deirdre, coming in behind Sibyl. "We got French pastries."

Deirdre did not look like hell. She didn't even look pregnant. She was willowy and ethereal, with flawless skin and huge, smoky gray eyes. Sibyl looked gorgeous as well. Her thick, curly hair was so deep red it was almost crimson, and her eyes above her high cheekbones were a shade of warm brown that matched her hair exactly. Soaking wet and without a trace of makeup, both of them would still have been beautiful women.

"Sorry about the mess," I said lamely. They didn't seem to register the comment. Sibyl set her bag down on the kitchen counter and began to pull out a variety of baked goods. Deirdre was carrying a large bottle of apricot nectar. She found the drinking glasses and filled three of them.

"Here, Martha," she said. "Try this. It was the only thing I could keep down for three weeks."

I was a little dazed. I took the glass obediently and tried a sip. Surprisingly, it tasted good.

"You were morning sick, too?" I ventured.

Deirdre rolled her enormous eyes. "Don't get me started."

"She just hit fourteen weeks' gestation yesterday," said Sibyl. "The nausea generally trails off after twelve weeks." She found a plate and began to arrange pastries on it. There were muffins, croissants, rolls, cookies, brioches. Sibyl had obviously been determined to find foods I could eat.

"Actually, this pregnancy hasn't been all that bad," said Deirdre, "compared to my first one. Now, *that* was disgusting. Sick as a cow, the whole nine months."

They carried the food and juice to the table that served John and me as both desk and dining room. I followed them, feeling a little strange because of the fact that this didn't feel strange. I wasn't used to inviting people into my apartment. I had made some great friends during my undergraduate days, but most of them had moved away from Boston. It had been much harder for me to form friendships since I started my doctoral training. Motherhood had made me the odd person out among my classmates; they were polite and kind to me but understandably less than fascinated by the details of my life as a nursing mother. I would show up at class after a night in the emergency room, where Katie had been put through a battery of hideously painful tests to determine the cause of some raging illness, and pretend that I really cared about the contrast between Karl Marx's view of historical necessity and Max Weber's. I would discuss Durkheim's theory of social contagion with my classmates during seminars, faking intellectual passion the way a frigid woman fakes orgasm, while I was actually worrying about teething pain or the need to baby-proof my bedroom. I had done this so often, under such intense conditions, that I had forgotten what it felt like to talk easily, freely, without any camouflage.

Sibyl and Deirdre were obviously used to communicating in this disarmingly open way. As I joined them at the breakfast table and picked out a brioche to chew, I watched and listened cautiously. They were intelligent and accomplished women, but neither of them displayed any of the interaction patterns I'd grown used to at Harvard. There was no sense of competition, no feeling that I was being judged and found either inadequate or threatening. Instead there was relaxed frankness, and a kind of warmth I had almost forgotten could exist. I didn't know how to respond to this. It made me nervous.

"You look better, Martha," said Sibyl as she refilled my glass of apricot nectar. "I'm relieved. Yesterday I thought I was going to have to haul you over to the hospital. Or maybe the morgue."

"I feel much better," I said, still awkward with gratitude. "Thanks to you."

Sibyl waved a hand dismissively.

"You're sorta thin, though," Deirdre observed as she bit into a croissant.

"Well, you should talk," I said. "You look about as pregnant as the Swan Princess."

"Mmm." She nodded, swallowing some croissant. "It's all the barfing. I'm not kidding, I could teach bulimia lessons. But now that I'm not as nauseated, I'll make up for lost time. I gained about a thousand pounds with my first baby, sick as I was."

"Isn't there something they could give you guys for the nausea?" said Sibyl. "Have you asked your doctors about it?"

Deirdre snorted. "Oh, yeah, a lot they care. They'd rather have you starve to death than take a Tylenol."

I nodded in agreement. "I think the Harvard doctors are afraid that if they give you permission to take a drug and something goes wrong with a baby, they'll get sued for malpractice."

"Doctors," said Sibyl, shaking her head. She launched into a series of medical anecdotes that had me laughing out loud for the first time in weeks.

The conversation flowed smoothly on to some other topic, and then another and another, all of them quirky, funny, engaging. I sat there cautiously, like someone who had suddenly been transported from Antarctica to a beach in Tahiti. Neither Sibyl nor Deirdre showed a trace of the snobbery I have often seen in beautiful women, nor was there any of the professional puffiness that had grown so familiar to me. Sibyl is a writer, Deirdre a musician, and they are both exceedingly good at what they do, but they spoke about their work the same way they discussed their stretch marks, without either conceit or false modesty. I found myself relaxing as if I had known them for years.

Looking back on that morning, I realized for the first time how lonely I had become. Harvard had slapped me in the face often enough to make me carefully self-concealing in any social interaction, and since I had become a mother, I had hardly spoken to anyone but John about anything that really mattered to me. With John in Asia, I felt as alone as if I were locked in a space capsule.

Of course, I had Katie, but that is not the same as having adult company. One of the great myths of our society is that when women are left with small children, they are not alone. The truth is that a mother left with babies is far more alone than she would be without them; every bit of energy, attention, protectiveness, and care she might use to meet her own needs must first be directed toward the needs of her children. That's why the Bible always laments the fate of "those who are with child and those who give suck" in the middle of war and disaster. The authors of the Good Book knew perfectly well that a woman alone can run, fight, or hide, but a woman with babies is toast.

I didn't think all this through as I talked to Deirdre and Sibyl over apricot nectar. I only knew that I was experiencing a strange melting sensation, that my control of my own image was beginning to get sloppy, and that it felt dangerously good. When Katie woke up and Sibyl immediately went to care for her, I was dismayed to find that, for the second time in two days, I couldn't help crying in front of someone. It was just that I could hear Sibyl and Katie laughing, and the thought that someone so loving was taking care of my daughter made it impossible to control the tears. At first Deirdre chatted on, diplomatically pretending not to notice, but when I had to wipe my eyes on the sleeve of my bathrobe, she fell silent.

"I'm sorry," I said, half-smothered with embarrassment. "I just . . . I don't know how to thank you. I can't figure out why you and Sibyl are doing this. I didn't do anything to deserve it."

Deirdre watched me for a moment in silence. "I don't know how much Sibyl has told you about me."

I squinted at her. "Nothing."

"Mmm," she said, nodding. After a pause, she went on. "I'm on my second marriage," she said. "My first husband was Mr. Perfect—handsome, charming, successful. He was also completely psycho. Someday

I'll tell you more about it. Right now, all you need to know is that I didn't have a clue who I'd really married. He started acting strange the moment I said, 'I do.' The longer we were married, the crazier he acted. After a few months, I started getting really scared. I left him when I was three months pregnant."

I stopped crying and looked at her more closely. She was as unruffled as ever.

"When I ran away, I was sick—sick like you are now. I was also a complete emotional wreck. Couldn't eat, couldn't sleep. I ended up in the hospital."

In the other room, I could hear Sibyl and Katie singing "Itsy Bitsy Spider."

"I thought I would die in that hospital bed," said Deirdre calmly. "My life had fallen apart."

"I'm so sorry," I said, feeling even more embarrassed to be making such a fuss about my own situation.

Deirdre shrugged. "It was a while ago. Things are good now. But I want to tell you about something that happened while I was in the hospital. It was late, after visiting hours. I had an IV in my arm, which was a good thing, because I couldn't even try to eat or drink. They gave me a cup of water, but I was too weak to pick it up. And I couldn't stop crying."

She noticed that I had finished my brioche and pushed the plate with the pastries toward me as she talked.

"Sometime around midnight, a nurse's aide came in to mop the linoleum in my room. She was a little woman—couldn't have been more than five feet tall—with gray hair and dark brown skin. She could have been Mexican or Filipina or Egyptian, for that matter. I don't know. But she didn't speak English. She kept looking at me as she mopped, watching me lie there crying. Then she said something in a language I didn't understand. She put her mop in her bucket, went into the bathroom, and came back with a basin of warm water and a clean cloth. And then she began to wash me."

Deirdre touched her own forehead, then each of her wrists as she spoke.

"She cleaned my face, then my hands and arms, and then lifted the blanket to wash my feet. The whole time, she kept talking to me in this language I didn't understand. But I knew what she was saying."

Deirdre inclined her head toward the other room, where Sibyl was making soft cooing noises as she got Katie dressed. It took me a second to figure out what she meant, and then I suddenly understood. She was talking about the soothing, singsong language mothers speak spontaneously when they talk to babies. Baby talk is found in all nations, all cultures; it is the original Mother Tongue. It translates across any language barrier because it is more about music than about words; the sounds themselves, not their meaning, give comfort and support.

Deirdre reached out one hand and laid it over mine. "That's why I'm here," she said. "I have a debt to repay."

By this time, of course, you could have used me to irrigate the North Forty.

"That sounded wrong," said Deirdre. "I mean, I did come today to repay my debt. But I'll come back because I like you." And she flashed me a quick, gorgeous smile as Sibyl carried Katie in to breakfast.

⌢ This was my first tentative, wary encounter with one of the greatest gifts I would receive from Adam: the understanding that the word *mother* is more powerful when it is used as a verb than as a noun. Mothering has little to do with biological reproduction—as another friend once told me, there are women who bear and raise children without ever mothering them, and there are people (both male and female) who mother all their lives without ever giving birth. The bad news is that not all of us have the good fortune to be born to our real mothers, or to stay with them as long as we need them. The good news is that, while mothers are often in short supply, mothering is not. Against all odds, despite everything that works against it on this unpleasant, uncomfortable planet, mothering is here in abundance. You can always find it, if you're smart and know where to look.

Of course, while I was expecting Adam, I ended up being mothered even though I didn't have a clue where to look. Not only did I fail to go out and find people to mother me through that difficult time, I actually tried to keep them away when they showed up on their own. You have to let down your defenses in order to be mothered, and after seven years in a culture obsessed with academic achievement, my defenses were just about the only parts of my personality I had left. Whatever force it was that brought Sibyl up to my apartment, and made her return with Deirdre the following day—and the day after that, and the day after that—was also loving enough to make sure I was too sick to send them away.

I'm not sure what that force was. For a while, after that wild year, I tried to assign a name to it: serendipity, good fortune, God, destiny. If you want to call it any one of those names, you are welcome to do so, but at this point I can't say I know for sure. Whatever it was, I suspect that, even then, Adam was working for it. I wouldn't be at all surprised to learn that he had picked out Sibyl and Deirdre, chosen them to show up at my apartment. It sounds like something he would do.

8

⤸ Sibyl and Deirdre fortified me with enough apricot nectar and loving-kindness to keep me out of the hospital until John returned from his first trip. Unfortunately, he brought some uninvited visitors with him.

We'd known when John took the Singapore assignment that he would be exposed to some weird germs. We had lived in Southeast Asia for a year right after we were married (I finished my junior year of college at a Chinese-speaking research center in Singapore) and had suffered from a number of strange diseases. One of them made our eyelids go all scaly, so that it looked like we had little lizards perching next to our noses. Another caused our ankles to quiver independently from the rest of our bodies. I had a few embarrassing gynecological problems that required visits to the Clinic for Wormen [sic]. Mostly, though, the Asian germs we'd picked up, and the new ones John caught and brought back to Boston in 1987, caused the same general assortment of symptoms that sweep through the United States every flu season. Body aches, headaches, toothaches, hair aches, heartaches—you name it, in 1987, we ached it. Exhausted, stressed, and constantly shuttling around the entire globe, John was a virtual petri dish for the transportation of aches.

The physical problems he brought home that November included a severe intestinal virus, an antibiotic-resistant sinus infection, and lice. I contracted all of these about five seconds after he walked through our apartment door. After a two-week separation, I didn't give a damn about the infectious aspects of kissing. John's mouth tasted like mentholated throat lozenges and cough syrup, but it also tasted like him, so I didn't care. His taste reminded me of butternuts, which grew in abundance around my house when I was a kid. They're similar to walnuts, but wilder, with an aftertaste like the air in a forest during a rainstorm. I inhaled John's scent, with its mixture of woodsiness and medication, like a glue-sniffing addict sucking up a fix. It was the only smell in the world that didn't make me want to throw up.

By midnight, however, the intestinal virus had taken hold, and I was in the throes of truly record-setting stomach upset. I spiked a high fever and became delirious. I kept swimming around in the bedclothes, making strange muttering noises, trying to curse God and die like Job's wife advised him in the Bible. Eventually, John became concerned enough to take me over to the University Health Services emergency room. I barely remember getting there. The doctor on call peered into my eyes and ears, and informed us that I was severely dehydrated and needed intravenous fluid.

Then, suddenly, the doctor's eyes opened wide. She looked at me as though she were seeing something wondrous and rare. Actually, she wasn't looking at all of me. Just my arms.

"Janice," said the doctor softly. Then she called, a little louder, "Oh, Janice! Come here, please!" She kept her eyes fixed on my forearms as though she had spent weeks of unsuccessful whale watching and they were two baby belugas.

Nurse Janice appeared in the doorway of the small examination room. "Yes?" she said.

"Look at this," said the doctor. She reached out and picked up my left hand.

The nurse looked, and her eyes widened. "Oh, my," she said reverently.

"Go get Brenda," said the doctor.

At this point I was vaguely glad they seemed to like my arms so much, but I had no idea why. Now I know.

You see, I have these very large veins. Even now, as I type these words, my computer screen casts a blue-gray glow across my hands and wrists, throwing those veins into sharp relief. They are, indubitably, very large— and I am no longer pregnant. When any woman is pregnant, her veins get bigger to handle the increased blood volume. That morning in the emergency ward, my arm veins rivaled your average garden hose in diameter and fluid capacity. You could have driven a bus through them. I was, of course, aware of this, but I did not know what it meant to the medical staff at University Health Services. Nor did I understand the significance of sending for Brenda.

It turned out that Brenda was a brand-new nurse, just finished with her R.N. degree, embarking on an entire career of piercing people's skin with sharp objects. To do this skillfully requires a good deal of practice. This is especially true for inserting IV's, which are much thicker than syringes and have to be threaded a fair distance into a vein so that fluids can be pumped through them. To learn this skill, nurses practice a lot, first on citrus fruit, and then on each other. Yes, each other! I have a wonderful sister-in-law who used to come home from her nursing classes with track marks like a heroin addict. As far as I'm concerned, she and everyone like her should be granted sainthood immediately, without further discussion. But nurses only have so many veins to offer up to collegial experimentation, so they are always on the alert for patients with really big veins. Persons like little old pregnant *moi*.

When Brenda came in, she could hardly contain herself. She and Janice and the doctor all spent a minute clucking admiringly at my vast veins. Then they whipped out the IV equipment, and Brenda gave it her best shot (so to speak). She was really good at getting the needle through my outer layer of skin and into a vein but had considerably more trouble threading it through the vein without punching it out the other side. She punctured three veins in this manner, all the time horrified to think she was hurting me.

This ushered in an era of my life I call the Pincushion Period. I would require rehydration every few days for the rest of my pregnancy, and every beginning nurse at Harvard University Health Services would get a shot at me (so to speak). Years after Adam was born, a friend gave me a recording of a song about a woman who was pregnant and frightened and lost. As I listened to it I felt a great wave of sadness wash through me—not an intrusion of grief from outside but a release from within. Someone understood how I had felt. I was sitting alone in my living room, listening to the song and crying, when I felt a sharp pain in my right forearm, as though I'd been stung by a bee. I looked down to see that one of the veins in my wrist—the biggest one, which was always the first target of the neophyte nurses—had broken open. It was bleeding under my skin, forming a maroon bruise that spread slowly. There is research that indicates individual cells might be able to learn, to remember, and to replicate experience. I have no doubt that as I listened to that song, the cells in my enormous vein were telling their humble story as best they knew how.

⇒ At the time I actually got all those IV's, I never minded the slight pain in the arm that came with them. On the contrary. I came to love those beautiful clear bottles of glucose solution from the moment that Brenda finally succeeded in hooking me up to one. As the liquid dripped into my bloodstream, my vision slowly cleared. The extreme weakness of dehydration was replaced by something close to a sense of well-being. Best of all, I didn't have to eat or drink. Forcing myself to take in nourishment was a constant struggle, and having calories and fluids pumped directly into my veins was like having a baby-sitter for the fetus. I lay back and relaxed, grateful beyond measure for medical science and its practitioners.

It takes a long time to funnel three quarts of liquid into a human vein, even a very large one. After making sure I was comfortable, Brenda, Janice, and the doctor left me to rest and absorb glucose solution on my own. I fell into a deep, healing sleep.

And then I began to dream.

If it were possible to convey in words the true experience of a dream, we probably wouldn't need dreams in the first place. They come from someplace beyond our rational and verbal minds, and are by nature indescribable. The dream I had that day in University Health Services is even harder to convey than most. But I'll try.

I was sitting by a wooden table, in a room filled with slanting light from a half-shuttered window. Strewn across the table were hundreds of documents, all yellowed with age and torn by rough handling. I felt desperate and overwhelmed. I knew for some reason that I was supposed to find something of great significance in the pages, but I had no idea where to look. As I searched through the stacks of paper, the atmosphere around me seemed supercharged, volatile, brimming with the anticipation of some immensely significant event. My compulsion to prepare for this unknown occurrence was almost frantic.

Eventually I became aware that I was not alone. I looked up from my papers and saw, sitting across the table from me, a young man. At least the form of a young man. I had the sense that this person was in fact ageless, but from his appearance I would have taken him to be in his mid-twenties. I remember this even though I have no memory of what he actually looked like.

"Here," he said, and reached across the table to hand me a piece of paper. His voice was incredibly resonant and gentle, so much so that it brought tears to my eyes. I knew immediately that the page he gave me was the one I had been looking for. It contained exactly the information I most needed to know. Nevertheless, I reached out to take it with great reluctance—no, make that terror. It scared the bejeezus out of me to open my hand and close it on that single sheet of paper. The intensity of my fear was matched only by the intensity of my desire to see what was written there.

The memory of reading that letter is much fainter now than it was later that night in our apartment, when I wrote down everything about the dream I could recall. Even so, ten years later the images remain incredibly vivid in my mind. The letter was written in characters I had never seen before, in a language I did not know. However, I could understand it immediately, and in fact it seemed a much clearer language than English. Reading it felt like coming home to my native country after many years in alien territory. The words of this unknown tongue had been laid down in a firm, graceful hand, and they shone. Literally. A brilliant golden light, like the reflection of the setting sun over water, flashed and sparkled from every mark and line. It was as though the pen had not put down pigment but scraped away material reality to reveal something inexpressibly beautiful shining beneath it. As I read the letter, I felt a deep comfort trickling into my heart the way the glucose solution was trickling into my veins.

Brenda woke me by setting one soft hand on my shoulder. I had been asleep three hours, and the IV drip had done its work. I felt much, much better. The virus was on the wane, my tissues were plump with beneficial fluids, and I could stand up on my own. But besides these physical blessings, and far beyond them, the echo of the dream remained with me. I felt as though I had been bathed in light. Brenda left me to get dressed, and for a few minutes I sat quietly, turning over the dream in my mind as though it were some complex and exquisite piece of jewelry. The visual details were still breathtakingly vivid, but to my great frustration, I couldn't remember anything about the content of the letter—not a word, not a phrase. However, there were things I knew after having that dream that I had not known before. I was irrationally certain of three things: that the ageless young man across the table from me was the fetus I carried in my womb; that this being loved and respected me as his equal; and that there was "something wrong" with the baby.

I put my clothes on very slowly. For weeks now strange emotions and impressions had swirled around inside me like some strange drug. I was constantly feeling things I neither expected nor understood. As I pulled on my shoes, I tried to dismiss my new irrational beliefs, especially the one about the baby's having some kind of problem. Ridiculous, I thought defensively. Just the kind of nightmare any pregnant woman would have after sucking up pizza for twelve hours. The strange thing, though, was that I didn't feel as if I'd had a nightmare. The comfort that had settled into my very core as I read the young man's letter had not dissipated when I awoke. It had been a good dream. A very good dream.

⌐   Brenda and Janice were manning the nurses' station when I went to check out. They seemed very pleased to see me on my feet, with my skin all pink rather than dead-carp white. I thanked them for their help as I gave them my Harvard ID card and signed release papers. When I turned to go, something made me hesitate.

"Um . . . ," I said awkwardly. "I was wondering—do you know if a virus like the one I just had—you know, an ordinary stomach virus—could cause some kind of problem this early in a pregnancy?"

Brenda looked at Janice, who had more experience. Janice furrowed her brow.

"Oh, I really don't think so," she said, in that crisp, firm voice nurses use to keep patients from delusions of catastrophe.

"Because," I went on, "I know what can happen with German measles, and toxoplasmosis, and things like that."

"Yes, of course," said Janice kindly. "A lot of things can go wrong. But I don't think you have anything to worry about. Eat right and take care of yourself, and the baby will probably be just fine."

For some reason, I couldn't seem to let go of the subject. "If something were wrong with it—the fetus, I mean—when could I tell? How would I know?"

This time, Brenda got the courage to speak up. "Usually, when something is wrong, the pregnancy miscarries," she explained. "Other things we don't know about until the baby's born—unless we test for specific problems."

"So," I said slowly, "what kinds of tests are available here? What do you test for?"

Janice took up the thread again. "Aside from the usual checkups, where we listen for the heartbeat and so forth, there are several kinds of tests available. We can screen for some with ultrasound, some with blood tests. There's always amniocentesis, where we draw amniotic fluid from the uterus and analyze fetal cells. And then there's chorionic villi sampling—that's where we analyze a bit of tissue from the umbilicus, and it can be done a lot earlier than amniocentesis. But those aren't standard procedures. For a woman as young as you are, with no family history of birth defects, they're all optional."

I thought about this for some time.

"I don't think your insurance would cover most of the procedures, anyway," Janice went on, probably wondering how to get rid of this strange, loosely clad, barnaclelike creature that had attached itself to her nurses' station.

"Which ones *would* it cover?" I asked.

"Well, the blood tests. AFP, if you want it."

"AFP?"

"Alpha-fetoprotein," she explained. "It's a waste product from the fetus. If there's a great deal of it in the mother's bloodstream, it can indicate spina bifida."

"Okay," I said. I remembered that they had asked if I wanted that test when I was carrying Katie. I had declined, since my risk factors were so low. But now, something paradoxically warm and terrifying was pushing at my consciousness. I gave Brenda and Janice a final word of thanks and took the elevator to the third-floor obstetrical department. Before I left the clinic, I wanted to make sure that I had signed up for every single prenatal test covered by my insurance.

Ten years later, I still believe that Adam suggested this himself, as a way of helping me prepare to become his mother.

⌐ Right now, from the room directly beneath my office, I can hear Adam bellowing at his older sister for taking a can of Coca-Cola away from him. She took it because she knows that's what I would do if I were downstairs. I don't give Coke to my kids, but I keep a secret stash of it for a writer friend of mine. Adam had just located my latest hiding place. He had guzzled one can and was on to his second when Katie caught him. After that one Coke, we can expect Adam to get totally wired on sugar and caffeine, and spend several soulful hours strumming away on his guitar and singing love ballads about his girlfriend, Lonnie. (The first time I heard him singing, through the door of his bedroom, I thought he was having a seizure. I almost called 911 before I dared to go into the room. When I opened the door, there he was with a small plastic guitar, serenading the moon with sounds like a cat being run through an electric lawn mower.)

What I'm trying to say here is that Adam is not some oracular phenomenon, like Jesus in the Temple astonishing the scholars with his insights, or that kid in Seattle who was recognized by Tibetan monks as the latest reincarnation of a high lama, or even Shirley Temple, who could really dance. He's just a kid with a boyish enthusiasm for tormenting his sisters and a voice like one of the Billy Goats Gruff. Most of the time. I tell that part of the story to strangers and friends alike. I generally keep quiet about the fact that, every now and then, something different shows through Adam's retarded-child facade. It glints like the light that shone from the lines of that dream letter I read ten years ago, and it can take your breath away.

When Adam was three years old, I began to lose hope that he would ever communicate verbally. His inability to speak was terribly frustrating for him, and it just plain broke my heart. I worked with him for hours, doing the exercises the speech therapists had taught me, having no success whatsoever. Sometimes Adam made random sounds that could be force-fit into words, but not with any degree of honesty. I had to face it: the kid couldn't talk. Not at all.

One day, after hours of unsuccessful therapy, I hit a low point. I took my children to the grocery store and offered them all bribes to keep quiet—I was too tired and discouraged to enforce discipline any other way. I told them they could each pick out a treat from the candy stands next to the checkout counter. When we got there, Katie chose a roll of Life Savers and Lizzie a chocolate bar. Adam, who seemed to understand everything I had said even though he couldn't speak in return, went over to a basket of red rosebuds and pulled one out.

"This is what you want?" I asked incredulously.

He nodded.

"No, honey, this isn't candy," I said, putting it back and turning him toward the rows of sweets. "Don't you want candy?"

Adam shook his small head, walked back to the bucket, picked out the rose, and put it on the counter. I was baffled, but I paid for it. Adam took it gravely as the girls unwrapped their candy. He held the flower with both hands all the way home. When we got there, I was immediately engrossed in putting away the groceries and forgot all about his strange request.

The next morning I awoke to find sunlight streaming through my bedroom window. John had already left for the day, and I could hear quiet babbling coming from Lizzie's room. As I yawned and stretched, I heard Adam's small feet padding down the hallway toward my bedroom. He appeared at the door with the rose, which he had put in a small crystal bud vase. I looked at him in surprise. I didn't realize that he knew what vases were for, let alone how to get one down from the cupboard, fill it with water, and put a flower in it.

Adam walked over to the bed and handed the rose to me. As he held it out, he said, in a clear, calm voice, "Here."

It had been years since I had thought about my dream at University Health Services, years since I had heard the incredible gentleness in the voice of the young man who had sat across the table from me—the same voice I had just heard coming from my mute son's mouth. I stared at Adam, almost frightened, as the dream flashed into my mind. He looked back at me with steady eyes, and I knew what I had known—what I should have remembered—all that time: that his flesh of my flesh had a soul I could barely comprehend, that he was sorry for the pain I felt as I tried to turn him into a "normal" child, and that he loved me despite my many disabilities.

Then he turned around, his little blue pajamas dragging a bit on the floor, and padded out of the room.

9

◟ I don't think I realized quite how obsessive people can be about appearances until I began to talk to some of Adam's physical therapists, who started working with him when he was two weeks old. First of all, you must know that the people who spend their lives working with disabled children are the most accepting, loving, optimistic-but-realistic human beings you could ever meet. To them, no child, no matter how disfigured or inept, deserves anything less than unconditional acceptance. Adam's therapists probably don't know that I, with my three Harvard degrees and my relatively sound body, got more from their sessions with Adam than did Adam himself. As I sat watching them, feeling the kindness in the air around them, all the parts of me that I had sent to the Deepfreeze years before thawed and stretched and began to consider the idea that the world might not be altogether hostile.

This is not to say that Adam's therapists didn't make any judgments. They were, in fact, secretly appalled by some of the people they had met in their line of work. Two of them told me this one day when Adam was working out, trying to bulk up from nine pounds. (The workout consisted of things like grabbing for shiny objects, cranking his head back and forth to hear interesting sounds, and rolling around in a tub of dry beans.) The conversation turned to other children the therapists had worked with—specifically, those who were recovering from major surgeries demanded by parents who were dissatisfied with their children's appearance. The therapists had worked with children whose thighbones had been shattered and reconstructed to correct slight bowleggedness; others who had undergone plastic surgery to correct "defective" features that had not yet even formed; still others who were given up for adoption because of anomalies as minor as a harelip. The therapists were outraged by these parents' inability to see beyond the issues of appearance to the core, to the child as a human being.

You must bear in mind that these therapists had *chosen* to work with "different" children, while the parents in question had had the experience thrust upon them. I'm certainly not one to judge them. I've had a hard enough time learning to handle difference without discomfort, to look beneath the surface. I do feel sad, though, for parents who might have had an opportunity to learn a new way of seeing, to look into the magical part of life, and let it pass them by. Then again, it may be that not all disabled children can do this. Maybe it's just Adam himself. In his strange, not-quite-human way, he is constantly reminding me that real magic doesn't come from achieving the perfect appearance, from being Cinderella at the ball with both glass slippers and a killer hairstyle. The real magic is in the pumpkin, in the mice, in the moonlight; not beyond ordinary life, but within it.

Here's another "shopping with the kids" story. One day when Adam was five, I took all three of my children out to pick up a few household items. I parked the car, extracted my children (two from car seats), and began the process of herding them all into the store without getting killed by traffic. I had Lizzie by the hand, and the older children were following—at least until we reached the doorway. We were at someplace like Kmart, where they sell gardening goods. That morning the store was holding a sale on ornamental plants. Flowers and shrubs were lined up on benches and tables just outside the door. The display drew Adam like a moth to the flame. His eyes got round—well, as round as they ever get, considering—and he began to coo with delight.

"Come on, Adam," I said, steering Elizabeth over to an empty shopping cart. "Keep moving, keep moving, keep moving."

By the time I had lifted Lizzie into the cart, Adam had disappeared. I gave that weary sigh—the one you remember your own mother sighing, the sigh that is sighed at least once a day by every parent of small children—and went back a few steps to look for him. He was over by the gardening display, walking away from me.

"Adam!" I hollered, trying not to sound too much like a child abuser. "Come here! Get back here!"

He looked up and blinked.

"Come on!"

Adam shrugged and, with a lingering look at the gardening display, trudged over to my grocery cart. I had the two older kids grab the bars of the cart, as usual, and we headed into the store. Just then I felt a tap on my shoulder. I turned. A very tall, very craggy, very elderly man was standing behind me. He was wearing a baseball cap with the name of a cattle-feed company emblazoned on it. He had the huge, rough hands of a lifelong farmer.

"Excuse me, ma'am," he said, doffing the baseball cap. "I was wondering if you noticed what your boy was doing just now."

I felt a surge of apprehension. Adam had done some profoundly embarrassing things in his short lifetime. He had hidden his shoes in my mother-in-law's microwave, crammed crayons into the baby-sitter's heating vents to watch them melt, gone over to visit the neighbors, alone, wearing only galoshes and a bra. My bra. I couldn't imagine what he might have done in the brief time I'd lost track of him outside, but his creativity in these matters always went well beyond my imagination.

I answered the old man with a cautious no, trying to look harried and innocent.

The old man leaned down to speak softly in my ear. "Your boy," he said, "stopped to smell every single plant in that display outside."

"Oh," I said uncertainly.

"He didn't just smell the flowers," said the farmer. "He smelled the shrubs, too. He smelled every bush they have out there. I think he even smelled the dirt."

I blinked at him, not altogether sure I was getting the point.

"Come with me." The farmer turned and gestured. He seemed very pleased, almost boyish. I turned my shopping cart around, children still attached, and followed him.

We went outside to the gardening display, the old man leading. I caught up to him next to a row of ornamental juniper brushes. He was leaning over, his eyes closed, inhaling deeply through his nose.

"Smell this," he said, pointing to the juniper. Katie and Adam had already begun sniffing. I put my face close to the shrub and smelled it. It had a tangy, sharp scent, somewhere between citrus rind and sagebrush. The smell brought back a sudden flurry of memories from my child-hood.

"Huh!" I said.

"It's something, isn't it?" The farmer gave me a crusty grin. "Now try this one."

We went on smelling bushes for five or ten minutes, until we'd sniffed our way through the whole display. I was so relieved that Adam hadn't done anything illegal that I hardly even wondered why this gruff, practical-looking man was so invested in the whole thing. Adam and the girls thought it was wonderful; they snuffled through the rows of plants like happy truffle hogs. As far as I was concerned, the bushes beat Proust's madeleine hands down; if you want to stir your imagination and your memory, I recommend that you immediately locate and smell some shrubs—whatever kind grew in your neighborhood when you were younger and closer to the ground.

When we were finished, the old man straightened up to his full height and tipped his hat to me again.

"Things aren't always what they seem, are they?" he said.

"No," I agreed.

"It pays to look close," he said. Then he leaned over again, put his lips near my ear, and whispered, *"My boy's twenty-three."* Then he turned on the heel of one enormous boot and walked away.

Ah, I thought. No wonder. He's one of us.

That's the kind of life you lead when you have an Adam around. Oh, of course it's not all lovely epiphanies. For every old man who invites you outside to smell the bushes, there are at least three obsequious sales-people who will congratulate you on having "such cute little girls," while they look awkwardly past the boy with Down syndrome, trying to pre-tend he isn't there. The prejudice, sometimes even hostility, can burn like acid. But along with this pain, Adam brought with him a sweetness that surpasses anything I ever felt before he was conceived. It comes from looking at the heart of things, from stopping to smell not only the roses but the bushes as well. It is a quality of attention to ordinary life that is so loving and intimate it is almost worship.

⌐ At Harvard, of course, I had learned to pay attention to very different things. The importance of prestige is so overwhelming in that culture that people hardly look at each other, let alone their environment. The attention goes to appearances: appearing successful, appearing smart, appearing utterly and absolutely unlike a retarded child. I began to notice this when I was pregnant with Adam, months before I had any solid evidence that there was anything "different" about him. Maybe his way of seeing, the depth of his appreciation for life, seeped from him into my bloodstream, or maybe it was the immediate proximity of his soul that affected mine. Whatever the reason, things began to look different.

It was mid-November and the few remaining leaves rattled on the trees. I welcomed the winter chill, since icy air helped keep my mind off the nausea. I breathed it carefully one day as I waddled over to William James Hall (known to the intelligentsia as Billy Jim) to attend a class. I arrived a few minutes early and decided to use the extra time to visit a friend in the Psychology Department, one floor above the Sociology Department, where my class was held. My friend was in her lab, conducting an experiment that consisted of implanting wires into the brains of live rats, then making the rats swim around in a tub of reconstituted dried milk. She told me why she was doing this, but I have no memory of what she said. Maybe she was making soup. Whatever the reason, she had put the rats and the milk in a children's wading pool, the kind you fill up with a hose so that toddlers can splash around on a hot summer day. The tub was decorated with pictures of Smurfs. Smurfs, for those of you who are not culturally aware, are little blue people whose antics you may have observed on Saturday morning cartoons during the 1980s. I personally feel that the Smurfs were cloying, saccharine little monsters, but Katie adored them.

After chatting with my rat-molesting friend for a moment, I excused myself and headed downstairs for the seminar. There were seven or eight other graduate students in attendance, along with a couple of extra professors who had come to hear the latest twist on established theories. I felt the way I always did when I walked into a classroom at Harvard, that I had just entered a den of lions—not starving lions, perhaps, but lions who were feeling a little peckish. The people in the room were fearsomely brilliant, and I was always terrified that I would say just one completely idiotic thing, make one breathtakingly asinine comment that would expose me as a boorish, politically incorrect half-wit.

"Ah, Martha," said the course instructor, "we've been waiting for you."

I blushed. I had stopped at the rest room to blow a few chunks, and had been hoping that the class would start a bit late. I did not want to be the focus of attention.

"I'm sorry," I said. "I was upstairs in the Psych lab, watching rats swim around in a Smurf pool."

"I see," said the instructor. "Yes, I believe I've read about that."

A professor, one of the visiting dignitaries, chimed in. "How is Smurf's work going?" he inquired. "I understand he's had some remarkable findings."

"Yes," said a graduate student. "I read his last article."

There was a general murmur of agreement. It seemed that everyone in the room was familiar with Dr. Smurf, and his groundbreaking work with swimming rats.

It took me a few discombobulated seconds to figure out that everyone at the seminar assumed a Smurf pool was named for some famous psychological theorist. I guess they thought it was like a Skinner box, the reinforcement chamber used by B. F. Skinner to develop the branch of psychological theory known as behaviorism. Comprehension blossomed in my brain like a lovely flower.

"I think," I said solemnly, "that Smurf is going to change the whole direction of linguistic epistemology."

They all agreed, nodding, saying things like "Oh, yes," and "I wouldn't doubt it."

I beamed at them, struggling desperately not to laugh. It wasn't so much that I wanted to mock these people. I was giddy with exhilaration, because after seven years at Harvard, I was just beginning to realize that *I wasn't the only one faking it.* I had bluffed my way through many a cocktail party, pretending to know all about whichever scholar or theory was the current topic of conversation. I had always wondered how I survived among the staggeringly intelligent people lurking all around me. Now I was beginning to understand.

"He's a good man, Smurf is," said the instructor solemnly.

And thus I learned that at Harvard, while knowing a great deal is the norm and knowing everything is the goal, *appearing* to know everything is considered an acceptable substitute. I pondered this great truth during the two-hour seminar. I was so buoyed up by it that I didn't pay enough attention to snorking up little bits of food in order to keep my nausea under control. I sailed right on into my next class, another seminar, confident that I could get through it without losing my lunch.

This was a mistake.

I still cringe when I think about that particular class period. I will continue to cringe about it until I am dead, and (who knows) probably for a long time thereafter. The course was Sociology of Gender, and the two instructors had managed to book just about every famous scholar in the field as a guest lecturer. I had been looking forward to hearing that day's speaker, a specialist on family structures and functions, for weeks. It was worth the wait. I'll always remember that scholarly gentleman. And I think it's safe to say that he'll always remember me. Oh, he doesn't know my name, and probably couldn't remember my face if his life depended on it. But I'm sure he can still recall that, right in the middle of this particular guest lecture, one student leapt to her feet, staggered toward the door, and passed out, collapsing in a heap so that she was lying with her lower body still in the classroom and her head and shoulders in the hallway. I have given many lectures myself since then, and I think it is safe to say that this kind of event would be hard to forget.

This was one fainting scenario in which the bystanders were not apathetic. Both course instructors were warm and considerate people. They immediately rushed to my assistance. (I don't think it's any coincidence that both these scholars left Harvard after a few years.) I don't remember how, but I ended up on a couch in the office of one instructor, Annemette Sørensen, confessing my pregnancy in a voice choked with shame.

"Well, there's nothing wrong with being pregnant," said Dr. Sørensen, "and if you're sick, you're sick. You might as well have been hit by a truck." I lay back on the couch, limp with embarrassment, warmed by her kindness.

"I'm better now," I said.

"How are you going to get home?"

I squinted at her. "I'm not going home. Class isn't over."

Sørensen pursed her lips, thinking. I could imagine her concerns; she hardly needed a repeat performance of my double-gainer to the classroom floor. To allay her fears, I took a long breath, pulled myself together, and sat up. Immediately, the hum in my ears increased to a loud buzz, the familiar green darkness flooded my vision, and I flopped back down again, briefly out like a light. When I came to, the second instructor, Lenore Weitzman, had joined Dr. Sørensen.

"We've got to get her home," she said.

"No, she says she wants to stay," Sørensen responded.

I tried to talk, but the best I could manage was an emphatic nod.

Dr. Weitzman looked at me as though I had just told her I intended to climb down the exterior walls of the building rather than ride the elevator.

"She's just pregnant," said Sørensen. In my seven years as a Harvard student, she was the only faculty member I knew personally who had actually given birth herself. "She'll be fine."

We reached a compromise. I spent the rest of that class period lying in the hallway next to the classroom. The door was left open so that I could hear what was going on. I had a notepad on the floor beside me, and I took notes in that strange, rambling hand you develop when your head is actually lying on the paper.

After class, a woman I didn't recognize asked if she could walk me home. She acted quite concerned, and the instructors, who seemed to have shouldered some responsibility for my well-being, were glad that I wouldn't be lurching the distance on my own.

My escort was another Ph.D. candidate. She was not in my department but had come to the gender seminar because of her passionate feminism. I, of course, thought of myself a feminist as well. Braced by the cold air and distracted by her companionship, I managed to keep up my end of an enthusiastic discussion of women's social roles. I liked my classmate very much.

When we got within eyeshot of the apartment building where I lived, I pointed it out and asked if she would like to come up for a little apricot nectar. I felt rather awkward doing this, but I wanted to thank her, and my breakfasts with Sibyl and Deirdre had made me bold.

She declined the invitation, smiling. Then her face became very serious.

"I wanted to walk you home," she said, "because I think it's time you stopped kissing up to the enemy."

I didn't have the vaguest idea what she was talking about, but I felt a chill in my gut. "Excuse me?"

The woman's face went so hard you could have chopped wood with it. "This crap about—what do they call it?—morning sickness. You know it isn't real."

I wasn't sure what to say. Morning sickness felt exceptionally real to me.

"Men have been telling women for centuries that it's hard to bear children," said the woman, as though she were repeating obvious facts to an Alzheimer's patient. "All that bullshit about the pain of childbirth, the 'delicacy' "—she said the word as if it tasted bad—"of pregnant women." She shook her head in frustration. "Bearing children is what women *do*," she went on. "There's nothing difficult or painful about it—unless you accept the party line. There is no such thing as 'morning sickness.' All of those myths were made up to justify denying women access to decent jobs and positions in society. And look at you—kissing butt like it's going out of style. Don't you think it's time to stop faking it?"

I just stood there with my mouth open. All those years of practice, and I had still let down my guard long enough to get another slap in the face. After a long time, I managed to say, "I don't think I can help it."

She went on in a voice that made me think of the feminist phrase "a pen dipped in anger," a voice that left no doubt that she put me in the same category with plague-bearing rodents.

"I don't care if you think you can help it or not," she said. "*Stop it!* It does not look right. It makes us *all* look bad. You're a dead weight on every woman alive. Just *stop it.*"

As I look back now, my strongest feeling about this woman is regret that I didn't kick her. At the time; however, I thought she was right. I was so drenched in shame for being pregnant in the first place, for not being a truly committed Smart Person like everyone else at Harvard, that it was very easy to accept the idea that my vomiting and fainting spells were psychosomatic.

"Um," I mumbled. "Okay, I'll try."

The woman rolled her eyes. "Yes," she said. "You do that." Then her face relaxed into a smile again, as though we had just been discussing the weather. "See you next week."

"Right," I said. "Next week."

I waited until she had turned and faded into the crowd along Massachusetts Avenue before I set out for home. Mind over matter, I thought, and held my head up high. I took the longest stride I could. Six inches, maybe seven. Damn. I was suddenly hugely self-conscious, and I felt a sense of panic, not so much because I truly believed I was ruining every woman's chances for a fair shot in life but because I knew somebody *thought* I was. "It does not look right," she had said. It does not look right. You do not look right.

I felt tears, those appallingly irrepressible pregnancy tears, forming in my eyes. And then, in the window of one of Mass Ave's many bookstores, I saw the cover of a children's book that bore the image of a small blue elf. It wasn't one of the Smurfs, but it reminded me of them.

"He's a good man, Smurf is," I said, imitating the professor who had said it earlier that day. A couple of passersby looked at me curiously but walked on. I felt the blossoming sensation in my chest again, the feeling of pulling back the petals and seeing the genuine heart of things. As I crept the final block toward the apartment building, I found myself actually smiling.

10

John hadn't begun to get over the jet lag from his second Asia trip before it was time for his third. He roamed our apartment at night, reading documents, grading papers, crunching numbers in the computer databases he was compiling for his dissertation. During the day, of course, we both went flat-out like racehorses in the stretch—well, anyway, John did. I was more like a hedgehog in the stretch. I had developed nausea associations with everything I was studying. I still get queasy when I see written Japanese, which I studied intensively that semester.

Even more distressing, my mental faculties were getting duller by the minute. I felt as though my brain had been replaced with a zesty blend of oatmeal and pond scum; I had lost the capacity for intellectual analysis, and my memory, which had once been reasonably good, seemed to have shut down operations altogether. After teaching—not just taking but *teaching*—an entire course on Caribbean culture, the only thing I can recall from the class is that the U.S. military referred to its attack on Grenada as a "predawn vertical insertion." And the only reason I remember this is that John and I took to using the phrase to describe the act that had gotten me pregnant in the first place.

Despite all of this, having John home made the world seem a decent place again. A good place. I once read the biography of a woman who described her husband with one sentence: "When he got home, the sun came out." Those were my sentiments exactly. Even as the days grew darker and colder, the time when John was home seemed bright. The first few snows actually struck me as rather festive. When John was there, it was easy for me to remember that Cambridge can be one of the loveliest cities on earth.

He left again on a Monday morning, early, having packed the refrigerator with foodstuffs of every possible variety in order to ward off another Death Spiral. On the outside of the door clung a set of magnetic letters, which John had bought for Katie. We had learned, much to our dismay, that two or three of the other Harvard-affiliated eighteen-month-olds in her day-care group were already reading. It was weird; they could read the labels on their Binkys while they were still using them. These children's parents had spent hours using flash cards to induce reading comprehension in their infants. John and I were amazed by this, and also much chagrined. We had the sick feeling that Katie had been inadequately trained, or perhaps (God forbid) simply wasn't up to the challenge of reading before the age of two. John had bought the magnetized alphabet to help launch her on the path to literacy.

I had thought that I would get used to letting him go, that each time would be easier than the last. Instead, it got harder. That day, after the apartment door closed and I heard the elevator pick John up, I went to the window and looked down at Mass Ave, hoping to catch another glimpse of him as he walked up the street to get a taxi. After a few minutes he came into view. He turned to look up at the window as I looked down at him. I waved, but he couldn't see me. Then he disappeared around a corner, and I went back to the bathroom.

I realized that I was fighting with a strange feeling. It was a sense of impending doom, a deep, terrible fear that had no basis in logic. I told myself it was normal that I should feel apprehensive. But this was something different. I searched my mind for a word to articulate the feeling. It took me a few minutes, and then I had it: *premonition.* I almost heard it, as though it were being whispered in my ear in four distinct syllables, *pre-mo-ni-tion.*

I shook myself like a wet dog and brushed my teeth. I didn't believe in premonitions, and besides, the sensation brought with it no instructions about how to avoid whatever it was I feared. I splashed cold water on my face and proceeded to my bedroom, where Katie was watching *Sesame Street.* All the other parents in Cambridge were flashing educational cards at their children, teaching them Greek and art history and organic chemistry, and Katie was becoming a one-and-a-half-year-old couch potato. I felt guilty about this, and worried about her educational prospects, but I was too weak-willed to train her at home. I hoped she was getting some academic skills at the day-care center. Katie looked up and smiled at me as I lay down next to her and closed my eyes.

Pre-mo-ni-tion. The word seemed to spell itself out in my head.

I put my hands over my ears, which was silly, because the word seemed to come from inside, not outside. It was only John's departure, I told myself. The suspicion that his plane was going to crash forced its way into my mind, and I began to sweat with the effort of not panicking. Half of me wanted to grab Katie, run outside, and catch John before he could find a taxi. The urge became more and more insistent. I shrugged it off, certain that he was already in a cab and well away from Harvard Square. But the feeling wouldn't go away. Even if I couldn't find John, the urge to leave the building was growing in me like a monsoon wind. I scowled and pushed back against it. I was too sick to go wandering through the city streets, especially with Katie in tow. Besides, it was snowing outside, and I was wearing nothing but one of John's T-shirts and a bathrobe.

I sat up and thumped myself on the head. I couldn't believe I was taking this thing seriously, arguing with myself, giving myself excuses for not rushing out of the building. With great effort, I wiped the pre-mo-ni-tion from my mind and lay down again.

I don't know how long I slept; probably not more than fifteen or twenty minutes. *Sesame Street* was still on when I was awakened by Katie's insistent little voice.

"Mommy," she said. "Red."

I peered at her through one eye. "What?"

"Red," she repeated. "Come see."

"What do you mean, Boofus?" I said. "What's red?"

Katie had turned away from me and was climbing onto the seat of a chair next to the window.

"One, two, three, four, five," she said. "Come see."

At that moment, we heard a sound like an immense duck quacking. It honked at regular intervals, shaking the walls with its volume.

"Oh, great." I sighed. "The fire alarm."

The fire alarm in our building went off every two weeks or so. When John and I first moved in, before Katie was born, there had been several weeks when it went off almost every night. Everyone in the building knew there wasn't any fire, but we'd all troop obediently down the stairs and assemble in the parking lot out back. It got so monotonous that people started bringing refreshments. It was the closest thing to neighborliness I had ever experienced in Cambridge. So when the alarm went off that morning, even after the pre-mo-ni-tion, I did not panic. I went calmly to the closet—walking, not running—and pulled on a sweatshirt and a pair of jeans. The jeans were getting depressingly tight around the waistline.

"Big duck!" I heard Katie say. "Big duck go quack!"

"Yes, honey," I said. "That's the fire alarm." She was still in her pajamas, the pink ones with the built-in feet. I went to get some clothes for her.

"One, two three, four, five," Katie counted again as I came back into the room carrying her clothes. I went to the window and put my arms around her.

"See, Mommy?" said Katie, pointing. Ten floors down, looking like bright toys in the morning light, was a cluster of fire trucks. Five of them.

I still refused to panic. Every fire alarm in a high-rise required at least one truck to show up. It was just a precaution. We residents of 1105 Massachusetts Avenue used to take down extra refreshments for the fire-fighters. True, I'd never seen five trucks at once. Maybe there actually was a real fire somewhere, a tiny fire, maybe a piece of bread lodged in someone's toaster oven. As I slipped a warm sweater over Katie's pajamas, I felt my fingers shaking. I took a deep breath and forced myself to calm down.

When Katie was dressed I walked, I did not run, to the closet for a pair of shoes. I slipped on some loafers and went to get my daughter, who was still looking out the window. I followed her gaze. The five trucks had spawned a whole congregation of firefighters, dashing around like ants whose hill was under attack. I didn't recall their acting this way in the past. I picked Katie up and was startled by how light she felt; I could tell that my muscles were getting juiced up with adrenaline. I shook my head in self-disgust and carried Katie—slowly, calmly, not running—toward the front door.

As I turned the corner into the living room, every one of my senses went on alert. The air felt warm and almost thick against my skin. I noticed a strange, toxic odor, faint but very pungent, that hurt my nose and left a foul taste in my mouth. Between the regular, deafening "quack, quack, quacks" of the fire alarm, I could hear the scuffling of feet in the hallway, a slamming door, a man's voice shouting. Looking down, I could see tentacles of thick, black smoke curling lazily upward from the crack beneath the door.

I tightened my grip on Katie, opened the door, and ran.

11

⤙ The door opened on a scene out of a disaster film. The air was billowing with noxious clouds of smoke. I could barely make out the shapes of my neighbors as they emerged from their apartments in pajamas and slippers. I saw confusion and panic on the nearest faces. I spotted a next-door neighbor running by.

"Where is it?" I yelled, trying to make myself heard over the fire alarm. "Where's the fire?" He just shook his head and kept running. Everyone on the floor was asking the same question.

I forced myself to think logically. The tenth story was too far up for fire-fighting equipment to reach, and there were no exterior fire escapes—no way to get down without going through the building itself. The amount of smoke made it clear that there was fire—a lot of fire— somewhere in the building. Fire goes up, I thought. It goes up. That meant that if the fire was below us, it would reach us soon. If it was above us, we were in less danger. Either way, staying on the tenth floor made no sense. I had to get Katie below the flames.

All of this registered in about six-tenths of a second. A Vietnamese family from down the hall came out of their apartment and rushed past me, yelling to each other. They dashed through the doors that led to the elevator.

"No!" I yelled, when I saw where they were going. "Not there! Take the stairs!" I wondered how they could push the elevator button every single day without noticing the signs that said, "In case of fire, do not use elevator. Take the stairs." I had a sudden image of what it would be like to be trapped in an elevator during a fire, choking on smoke, helplessly waiting for the flames.

The old woman for whom I had once run errands appeared in her doorway, face pale, eyes staring. She locked her gaze on me as other occupants ran past us.

"I cannot run," she said, in her thick Haitian accent. "I am ill, I cannot run!"

I remembered that she had asthma.

"Go into your bathroom!" I yelled. "Fill the tub with water and get in. Keep your head low. I'm going for help."

"Carry me!" she screamed, her eyes wilder than ever. I moved past her, toward the staircase door, and she reached out with one hand to seize my wrist in an amazingly powerful grip. "Carry me!" she pleaded. "I cannot run!"

"I can't," I said desperately. I could barely manage Katie; how could I carry her too? "I'll send help!" The smoke was getting thicker. I had to pry her fingers from my arm. I will never forget the look in her eyes as I pushed her hand away from me. It was the wild, desperate gaze of an abandoned child. I felt as though I were locking her in a gas chamber.

I ran to the door of the staircase and opened it, hoping to find less smoke inside. Instead, I was almost pushed backward by a dense, tarlike fog belching out of the open doorway. With my free hand I pulled the collar of my coat over Katie's head, trying to filter the smoke out of the air she breathed, and plunged into the blackness.

The darkness was absolute. I could not see Katie, could not see my own hair as it whipped across my eyes, could not see the walls or the floor or the stairs. I groped for the banister, found it, and ran down the first flight. Up until then, I realized, I had been holding my breath. I gulped for air. It was like breathing needles. Every cell in my lungs seemed to explode at once. I gagged and coughed, trying not to gasp, but it was impossible. My body felt as though I had not inhaled at all; I might as well have been immersed in a lake of poison. I turned the corner at the bottom of the first flight of stairs and ran down the next. Ninth floor.

I could hear Katie's ragged choking from beneath my coat. She had clamped her arms and legs around me like a frightened baby monkey. I felt a sudden surge of rage at the smoke. It seemed almost conscious, like a sentient evil searching for my child. I reached the bottom of another flight and turned again. Where was the fire? I had thought I would get below it quickly; there was too much smoke on the tenth floor to have come from much lower. Turn. Another flight. No light, no air. I remembered that most people aren't burned to death in building fires. The smoke kills them first.

The fire alarm was still blaring. It was incredibly loud. It shook my whole body with every blast. Between the deafening "QUACK QUACK QUACKS" of the alarm I could hear people screaming, dogs barking, feet running. I couldn't stop trying to breathe, though my lungs protested violently with every gasp. I was beginning to see spots and swirls of light behind my eyes, as though I had rubbed them much too hard. The air was getting hot. I realized that if I ran into the fire, I would not have enough oxygen to climb the stairs again. I reached the bottom of another flight. How many had I passed? I had lost count.

My lungs were almost numb, but now the rest of my body was beginning to cramp, sending stabs of pain the length of my arms and legs. I recognized the sensation from running wind sprints; it was the feeling of a muscle being pushed to move without oxygen. My limbs stiffened as the muscles filled with lactic acid. Another flight. Turn. Keep running. Stay on your feet and keep running.

Sparks of light were filling my field of vision now. I could feel my head lolling to one side. I slowed down slightly and was immediately hit from behind by people running past me. I clutched the banister to keep from falling. The arm holding Katie had gone rigid, like the claw of a dead bird. I began to weave slightly from side to side, and more bodies bumped into me. I held on tighter to the banister, pressed as close to the wall as I could, and kept going. It felt as though I had been in the stairwell forever. I was panting uncontrollably, but there was no air, no air, no air.

A woman screamed so close to my ear that I felt her breath, and she fell against me. I tried to scream myself, from rage and frustration and helplessness, but all that came out of my empty lungs was a strange, cawing sound. Another flight. Turn. There would be twenty flights, two to each floor. Where was I? And where in the name of God was the fire?

At the end of the next flight, when I let go of the banister and tried to turn, I fell sideways, pulled downward by Katie's weight. I grabbed for the wall, but my legs were like water. Then my foot came down on something soft and cylindrical, an arm or a leg. I could hear its owner choking and gasping as others tripped over him. I pitched to one side, fought for balance, and then felt my head smack hard into the wall. I fell.

It was anger that kept me from blacking out—anger not at my own situation but at this *thing*, this monstrous, evil thing that was trying to kill my daughter. I struggled to get to my feet, but I had lost all sense of which direction was up, where the stairs were located, anything that could have helped me get her to safety. Tears of rage ran down my face as I searched in my coat pocket for a mitten to tie over Katie's mouth and nose. If I couldn't go on, I would push her toward the stairs and hope that someone would find her, shove her, even kick her down the stairs. Anything but have her stay in that evil smoke to die of oxygen starvation. I found a mitten, but I was losing consciousness. I couldn't raise it to Katie's face.

It may only have been a second that I sat slumped against the wall, Katie whimpering and coughing in my arms, or it may have been as long as a minute. It seemed to be eternity. The anger still burned bright in my mind, but I couldn't move. My body had spent its last oxygen reserves, and now my brain was sputtering like a candle in a closed jar. The swirls of light grew brighter and stranger, and the sounds of the fire alarm, of people coughing and screaming, began to recede into a blank silence, far away from me.

I felt a hand on my arm. It felt like the neighbor lady's hand, the one I had torn from my arm a very long time ago, before I entered the smoke. It was bigger, though. Quite large, I thought vacantly, with my lamed and halting awareness. Probably a man. He was pulling on me. It was very unpleasant. My whole body was screaming for air—I was in enough trouble without panicky apartment dwellers pulling on me.

I felt the man's arm slide behind me, between my back and the wall, and he yanked me upward, hard, to my feet. Katie was still clinging to me. My right arm had stiffened around her so tightly I thought they'd have to bury us together. Save money, I thought distantly. Two people in one grave.

"*Three.*"

I blinked, trying to figure out who had said that. But everything looked the same, whether my eyes were open or closed. Three. Oh, yes, of course. Katie, and me, and the other one. I was carrying *two* babies.

I fell backwards, but the man had moved behind me so that I was leaning against him. He began to walk, pushing me along. I wondered how he could see in the smoke. The floor gave out under my feet, and I fell forward, but the man steadied me with his body, holding me upright. He was very strong. I felt my way down another step, and another, and another. I wanted to tell the man to put me down, to take Katie and let me be. I wanted to sit down again, go to sleep, give up.

Another step, and another, and another. I hit level cement and tried to turn, but the man wouldn't let me. He dragged me forward toward what I thought would be a wall—and then, suddenly, I was standing in the lobby of the apartment building on a bright December morning. The smoke in the stairwell was so thick that I could see nothing six inches into it. It was like a wall of sooty cotton batting. I took one huge gulp of air, like a swimmer emerging from a near-drowning, and the world rushed back into focus. The distant cacophony came back to surround me, the pinpoint stars were replaced by dazzling sunlight, the world felt real again.

I took another breath and went into a paroxysm of coughing. My lungs seemed bent on turning themselves inside out—anything to be rid of the gluey, pitch-black poison that had been rising up the stairwell as though it were an industrial smokestack. The coughing was so violent that I would have fallen again if the man had not braced me with his arm. I felt a strong hand on my back as I finally regained control of my breathing.

My eyes took a while to adjust to the sunlight, because of either the Stygian darkness in the stairwell or the lack of oxygen, or both. All I wanted to see was Katie. She was fine, not even coughing anymore, her white-blond hair dark with soot and her blue eyes wide.

"It's okay, honey," I told her, holding her more tightly than ever. "Everything is fine. We're okay." My voice came out in a strange, croaky whisper.

A firefighter in a heavy rubber raincoat rushed up to me, gave a brief glance at Katie, and said, "Ma'am, over here, please. Away from the building. Please."

I felt a gentle push from the hand on my back, and I staggered toward the far end of the parking lot, where my neighbors had already congregated. Most were in pretty good shape, if a bit rattled. They had come from the lower floors, and it had not taken them long to exit the building. The higher up the residents lived, the more blackened their faces. Those of us from the upper floors looked like coal miners, with smears of grit around our noses and mouths, where we had sucked in the smoke trying to breathe.

"What's going on?" I croaked as I got close to the group. "What happened? What's happening?"

A man whose name I didn't know, but whose face was familiar, turned to answer me.

"Food Shak," he said. "It blew up."

I stared at him. "The whole thing?"

"It was the refrigerators at the back of the store," said a woman. "Something caught fire, and then the whole thing just . . . went up. Didn't you hear the explosion?"

I shook my head, still dazed. My body was finally beginning to realize that I was out of danger. The adrenaline was seeping away from my muscles, and Katie was growing heavier by the second.

"It blew debris all the way across Mass Ave," someone else commented.

The same firefighter who had asked me to move ran past, toward the fire trucks.

"We've still got people in there!" he shouted. "I need a mask! Nobody goes in there without a mask!"

It was only then that I turned to search for my rescuer. I had never even seen him, and he hadn't spoken to me—except to say that one word, *three*, I wasn't even sure he had said that. The word seemed to have come from somewhere inside my head, although at the time I had been sure it was the man. I searched the crowd, looking for him, but there were so many firefighters and so much chaos that I knew it was hopeless. Unless he came up and introduced himself to me, I would never even know who he was. I let it go. My legs began to give out under me, as though I had just run fifty miles, and I carried Katie over to sit on the hood of a parked car.

During the next few minutes, as I sat panting and listening to the imbroglio around me, I learned that no one had been badly hurt by the fire, although many of us were suffering from smoke inhalation. The fire itself had blazed briefly through Food Shak, which was on the ground floor, and gone no further than that. The major problem was that the staircases were inadequately ventilated, so that they functioned as chimneys for the toxic smoke. Most of the people who had run down the stairs came from the first three or four floors and had simply held their breath for the few seconds it took them to get outside. Some upper-floor residents had taken the elevators. All of these people were just fine. The Vietnamese family, whose immolation I had imagined so vividly, were spending a pleasant morning breakfasting at the French café across the street, watching the firefighters douse the remains of Food Shak with their fire hoses. But I, with my unerring instincts, had waddled my feeble self into the most dangerous possible situation. I had taken the worse of the two chimneys, run further than anyone else, and because I was already sick, and carrying Katie, had probably inhaled more smoke than anybody in the building.

And that, sports fans, is how I made my Television Debut. A whole posse of cameramen and reporters rushed up and poked microphones in my face just a few minutes after my escape from the smoke, as I was wending my way toward the front of the building to see if the fire was out. They interviewed a lot of people that morning, but I was the one who was actually shown, for a few seconds, on the nightly news at six and eleven. The reason for this is that I looked and sounded about fifty times worse than anyone else in the vicinity. Now, I am not such a treat for the eyes on the best of days, but bear in mind that (1) I had just woken up; (2) I was covered with soot; (3) I was wearing glasses the thickness of the Berlin Wall, which made my head look strangely warped; (4) I had thrown up at approximately twenty-minute intervals for the previous two months, and was about to do so again; and (5) I had that pregnant glow about me, similar to the look you see on people who grew up in Chernobyl. I was also carrying Katie, with her blond, blond hair and her large, frightened eyes. Put it all together, and you can see why the TV newspeople were drawn to me like flies to a pile of dog feces.

The next day, to my profound humiliation, almost everyone I saw at Harvard would comment about my appearance on the news. They attempted to look concerned, but most of them couldn't help making that snorting sound people emit when they're trying not to laugh. The reporters in that parking lot had immortalized the one moment in my life when I looked absolutely as bad as I possibly could, and broadcast it to the entire known universe. It remains one of my life goals eventually to locate all copies of that news broadcast and burn them in a home incinerator I intend to build for the purpose. We each have our little daydream.

At any rate, the news broadcast was short. I had been on camera for all of fifteen seconds, croaking out some lame comment about how scary it had all been, while the pristine and comfortable Vietnamese elevator family smiled and waved to the camera from someplace just behind me. At least, I told myself, no one would ever see that film again. Memories do fade. By noon the next day I had decided that it probably wouldn't be necessary to kill everyone who had watched the news segment. Then, I happened to glance at a classmate's copy of the *Boston Herald*. The front page of the local news section was devoted to the fire at 1105 Mass Ave, and there were pictures. Large pictures.

The *Herald* photographer had caught me just as I burst through the smoke into the lobby and went into my coughing fit. My eyes were squinched tight behind those immense glasses, and my cheeks were puffed out as though I was pretending to play jazz trumpet. At first I was so dismayed by the way I looked from a distance that I didn't notice What's Wrong with This Picture. I stopped and stared at it, mesmerized by my total lack of photogeneity, and remembered the moment. I had been half-conscious, stumbling and limp, collapsing backwards against the strong, reassuring body of the rescuer who had found me and half-carried me out of the smoke. The picture in the *Herald* showed everything: my exhaustion, my fear, my confusion and disorientation. But there was one thing missing, one very large and important thing. As I gazed at the newspaper, replaying that instant over and over in my mind, the hair began to prickle along my arms and the back of my neck.

In the picture, there was nobody behind me.

12

﹂ I once saw a television special about a woman who was saved from falling off a cliff by some supernatural force, which she thought probably consisted of one or more angels. The woman and her fiancé had climbed a steep hillside to watch the sun set over the ocean. As twilight fell, they decided to take a shortcut back to sea level—an extremely short cut, as it turned out. The path they chose went almost straight down, and the rock face proved to be soft and crumbly. By dark, the couple were in serious trouble. The tide was coming in, and they were literally clinging to the fragile cliff by their fingernails. Then, just as the woman's strength gave out, she felt a strong, warm power lift her up, propping her against the rock. Aided by this mysterious force, she gradually made the climb to the beach, arriving safe and sound about fifteen minutes later.

In the meantime, her fiancé fell off the cliff and died.

After some of the things that happened to me while I was expecting Adam, I have no trouble believing this woman's story. I am quite ready to accept that Something helped her down that cliff, probably the same Something that got me through the smoke of the high-rise fire in Cambridge. But whatever the Something was, I can't fathom its motivation. As I watched the television special, I kept imagining what the woman's fiancé must have thought as he plummeted past his beloved, perhaps even seeing, as he went by, the angels who were gently transporting her to solid ground. If I had been in his position, I know what I would have thought. I would have thought, "So what am I, bat guano?" It would have been the last thing to go through my head, if you don't count the rocks at the bottom of that cliff. Perhaps the angels had a chance to explain their reasons to the deceased fiancé later, but I, for one, don't understand.

I get the same feeling when I look back on all the mysterious assistance I received during Adam's gestation. I don't know if other people from my apartment building had invisible helpers hauling them out of the smoke the day Food Shak burned. I doubt it. No one ever mentioned it. Perhaps, you may say, I was the only one who *really needed* paranormal assistance—but that logic doesn't work for me either. How many times a day does some poor hapless human *really need* a good supernatural protector and fail to get one? People are tortured and killed and raped and pillaged on a daily basis, and if there are angels in the vicinity, they apparently just sit around watching—wringing their ectoplasmic little hands, perhaps, but letting nature take its course.

A great deal of human energy, including mine, has been spent trying to figure out why some people get help from angels and some get lobotomized by flying debris from freak wheat-threshing accidents. Religious people always seem to have simple formulas to explain this. If you're very, very good, say the formulas, you can avoid the gods' disfavor and court their assistance. If you sacrifice a goat, you will be blessed. If it's the wrong goat—say, one with a gimpy foot—you will be smitten with a pox. If you join the right church, you will live long and prosper; if you leave it, you are consigned to eternal misery. Believe me, you don't grow up in Utah without hearing a great deal of this sort of reasoning. But none of the causal connections I have heard preached by any religion fits the facts as I see them. All I can say for sure is that whatever supernatural beings are operating around us, they are working from a priority list that is very different from mine.

Strangely enough, I have learned to trust them anyway.

Of course, all of these thoughts have occurred to me in the years since Adam came along. I didn't do much pondering of theological conundrums that morning in Cambridge. I wouldn't even begin to wonder about my invisible rescuer until the next day, when I would see the picture in the *Herald* and, for the first time, consciously articulate that something not merely unusual but actually paranormal was going on in my life. Immediately after the fire, I had more pressing issues to consider.

Breathing, for example. Even after I'd walked around in the clear, cool air for several minutes, my lungs felt needy, as though I were holding my breath, and whenever I inhaled, my chest felt as if it had been filled with crushed glass. To my relief, Katie was breathing more easily.

She said that her chest didn't hurt, although she did cough when the breeze blew wisps of smoke into our faces. I paced around, hacking like a tubercular cat, and the paranoia that had been haunting me since the beginning of my pregnancy began to pick up more steam than ever. I remembered statistics about the negative effects of tobacco smoke on human fetuses. It seemed possible that whatever blend of toxins I'd just breathed would have an even more destructive potential for the baby I was carrying. Perhaps this was the "something wrong" I had been anticipating. After worrying about this for a few minutes, I decided to seek a medical opinion.

Two ambulances were parked beside the fire trucks in the parking lot. A crowd of apartment dwellers, many in slippers and pajamas, had gathered around them. I carried Katie over to one of the ambulances and set her down on the feet of her little pj's. The burst of energy that got me down the stairs was long gone, and Katie seemed to have gained several hundred pounds. She kept a tight grip on my hand and the hem of my coat as I edged closer to the ambulance.

I got close enough to see that a line had formed in front of the ambulance doors. Inside the van, on the long benches that lined the walls, sat a group of my neighbors. They looked considerably worse than most of the people in the parking lot. Soot blackened their faces, and I could hear the rasp of difficult breathing as they inhaled oxygen through green plastic face masks. A paramedic was working his way through the crowd outside the van, lining people up to receive treatment in order of how severely they had been affected by the smoke.

"Excuse me," I said, raising my hand to get the paramedic's attention. He looked at me. "I just have a question," I said. "I'm pregnant, and was wondering if—"

But the paramedic wasn't listening anymore. He was shouting.

"Move back, move back!" he yelled to the people around the ambulance. "We've got a pregnant woman here! Move back!"

The crowd parted, clearing a path for me to reach the ambulance, as though the paramedic were Charlton Heston with a magic staff. At first I was confused, then embarrassed.

"Oh, no," I said. "No, thank you. I'm fine. I just wanted to ask a—"

"Right here, lady." Charlton Heston's voice was firm. He grabbed my arm with one strong hand and propelled me toward the ambulance. Katie pattered along behind me, and the paramedic noticed her for the first time.

"Okay, folks," he yelled to the people in the ambulance. "We got us an infant and a pregnant mother here. I'm gonna have to ask a couple of you to give up your seats."

"No," I protested. "Really. I'm fine. We're fine."

There was a space for eight people in the ambulance. As I peered inside, eight sets of traumatized eyes looked at me from behind eight green oxygen masks. And then, eight pairs of hands reached up to pull those masks free, every single one of them offering the precious oxygen to me and Katie. Charlton Heston took one from a pale, unhealthy-looking student, and one from a black man with a gray beard.

"Hell, I don't need that shit, anyway," said the older man as he climbed out of the ambulance. "I just need a cigarette." He grinned and winked at me as he went past. It was clear he was lying; his voice sounded terrible. I tried to thank him, but no sound came out of my own throat. I felt tears stinging in my eyes as the paramedic half-pushed me into the van, then picked Katie up and put her on the seat next to me. In all my time as a New England immigrant, I had never tested to see if there was kindness below the terse, tough exteriors of my fellow Bostonians. I had never known that such a thing was possible.

I tried to help Katie with her mask, but the paramedic pushed me aside and told me to put on my own. He tightened the elastic straps to fit Katie's small head, then talked to her soothingly while he showed her how to breathe into it. I held the soft green plastic to my mouth and took a cautious drag. My lungs still hurt, but the pure oxygen flowed almost tangibly into my blood, and the awful sense of suffocating began to lessen immediately. I fastened the straps around my head and I looked up. My six neighbors were all waiting politely, like guests at a banquet waiting for the hostess to pick up her fork, before they went back to breathing their own oxygen. No one said anything.

I put my hand up, supposedly to straighten my glasses, but really to hide the fact that, as usual lately, I was crying. I had done an immense amount of public crying since getting pregnant, probably more than I had in my entire life prior to that time. It wasn't that things were difficult—life was easier for me than it was for millions of people all over the world, and I knew it. The thing that got to me was the kindness, the thoughtfulness, the quiet and unassuming heroism of people like Sibyl and Deirdre and the neighbors who lived in my building.

Although it sounds crazy, I felt then, and still feel, that these small miracles always have clustered and always will cluster around Adam. When I was carrying him, I had the constant sensation that I was a kind of radio tower, within which Adam sat broadcasting some kind of signal to the world around me—not a verbal message but an unnamed energy, a sort of *goodness*, that drew out people's best selves and helped them connect with each other. Since Adam's birth, I have come to take this for granted. When he begins each academic year, I am always surprised that school personnel who aren't used to dealing with "different" children seem concerned, and sometimes even a little angry, at the thought of having Adam around. Even the wonderful teachers and principals who are used to children with disabilities don't act inordinately thrilled by Adam at first meeting. I have to remind myself that the mysterious force field around him takes a while to affect people. By the second or third parent-teacher conference, I introduce myself as Adam's mother and wait for their faces to light up. They always do. I have come to expect this, to see it as normal.

It's not that he does anything observably different from any other child. True, he is rather clumsy and slow, and almost everything he says sounds like the phrase "car wash" repeated several times backwards, but these are not the kinds of things that you would expect to create great outpourings of happiness in the people around him. And yet, the happiness always shows up. A friend of mine once observed, "Adam has angels like a dog has fleas. He came here with them, and the more time you spend around him, the more likely you are to get them yourself." That's as close as I can come to explaining Adam's force field, although, like the story of the woman on the cliff, there are many questions it leaves unanswered.

If you think all this sounds a bit odd, I must assure you that, to me, it *feels* a thousand times odder. This was especially true when I was pregnant, before I got used to the sensation. I was acutely aware of it as I sat between my neighbors in the ambulance, breathing air that any of them would have sacrificed for me, my baby, and my unborn child. I could feel the strange new energy radiating around me like the rings on the surface of broken water, showing me all the good in these people, helping them exercise it. I looked out the window of the van and reviewed the past several weeks, admitting to myself that I had felt this energy for some time, since before I knew I was pregnant. Then I shook my head hard and told myself not to indulge in such grandiose delusions. But the energy remained, and every time I began to relax, I felt it all over again.

I sat in the ambulance sucking up oxygen until the paramedics were convinced that everyone had escaped from the building. The last person to leave was my elderly, asthmatic next-door neighbor, who was carried out on a stretcher. She was a very rotund woman, and it eased my guilt a little to see that the four masked men carrying her were having considerable difficulty. If I'd tried to take her down the stairs with me, we'd probably both be dead.

After she was safely deposited in the other ambulance, the paramedics and firefighters began putting up barricades to keep people from entering the building. The fire was out, but the smoke was so full of dangerous and volatile chemicals that the entire place would be off limits to its inhabitants for three days while cleaning crews vacuumed the air. Please don't ask me how they did this, because I don't know. It sounds like something my mother-in-law would have done each and every day, right after she finished ironing the towels. All I know is that until the vacuuming process was completed, we of 1105 Mass Ave had to seek shelter elsewhere.

The parking lot began to clear as people resigned themselves to the situation and trickled off to the homes of friends or relatives, or to the school gymnasium where the paramedics had set up a temporary shelter.

The paramedics wanted to take me to the Harvard Medical Center, where doctors could test the levels of dangerous gases in my bloodstream. I was happy to comply. The more medical tests I could get, I reasoned, the more control I could exercise over the course of my own life and that of my child. It was my secular humanist's way of trying to sacrifice the right goat.

We spent a couple of hours at the medical center, where the nurses played with Katie and brought us both food. After they'd drawn some more blood and run a few tests, finding nothing alarming, the nurses offered to call a taxi for me. Now I had an interesting problem. I had left my apartment with nothing but Katie and the clothes I was wearing. I had no money, not even cab fare to the gymnasium where many of my neighbors were shacked up. Even if I could walk there, which did not seem probable, the thought of throwing up repeatedly in the communal rest room did not appeal to me. I could think of only one person to call.

Sibyl answered on the first ring. Fifteen minutes later her husband, Charles, pulled up with their daughter, Mie, in the backseat. Mie is almost exactly Katie's age, and the two of them looked at each other as though they had each struck solid gold. Within about twenty seconds, they were best friends, and would remain so until John and I moved away from Cambridge. Angels come in many shapes and sizes, and most of them are not invisible.

Sibyl, Charles, and Mie lived on the third floor of a quaint old mansion that shook every time a car passed outside, which was two or three times a minute. The structure had settled and slumped so much that there wasn't a single right angle left in it; the floor sloped gently downward, the ceilings sagged, and the walls bulged and rippled. The interior was beautiful; Sibyl had filled it with classic Shaker furniture and buffed the hardwood floors to a high shine. I have never been so grateful to be anywhere in my life.

It was afternoon when we arrived, and the pathetically weak winter sun was fading fast. I was not used to relaxing or having free time—when I wasn't caring for Katie or attending class, I was studying. But I had left all my books and my computer in the apartment, so there was little to

do except talk to Sibyl and watch Mie and Katie roll around like two puppies in a basket. I was simply amazed by how good this felt. Sibyl seemed
to know a great deal about prenatal medical care, and we spent a lot of
time discussing which tests I was going to request to make sure my baby
would be born healthy. I even told her about my gut feeling that there
was something wrong. She assured me that a lot of mothers had these
groundless worries. I nodded, but without conviction.

Katie and I slept on a makeshift bed that Sibyl put together in the living room. I don't know how much of her own work Sibyl had pushed
aside that day. She treated me as though she'd been dying to run a little
prenatal bed-and-breakfast. Some angels have red hair.

I lay in the darkness as Katie fell asleep beside me, feeling the house
shake whenever a car passed, listening to the scream of sirens from the
firehouse near Harvard Square. For every wail, there was somebody, not
so far from me, who was scared, hurt, dying, watching a loved one die. I
knew that John was probably still en route to Singapore, and against my
will I began to imagine his plane going down, smashing into the dark Pa-
cific a thousand miles from anywhere. My own mortality, the mortality
of everyone and everything I loved, leapt up and down before me in the
darkness, yapping and howling for attention. Every time I shut my stinging eyes, I was back in the dark stairwell, struggling for breath and balance. I began to tremble violently.

And then, just as I had in the smoke, I felt the touch of a hand. This
time, it rested gently on my back, and from it emanated a comforting
warmth that stopped my shaking and let me drift almost immediately
into an exhausted sleep. I didn't look to see where it had come from,
whose hand it was. I didn't even wonder. I seemed to know that touch
already, at some level far below my consciousness. The next day, stunned
as I was when I looked through that copy of the *Boston Herald* and saw
that my rescuer had not registered at all on film, some deep part of me
wasn't surprised.

13

John arrived in Singapore almost a full day after Food Shak had been reduced to a steaming charcoal shell. He had worked through the entire journey, reading and writing analyses of various business data for the Singaporean client. He called me from the Tokyo airport, where he changed planes, but of course I wasn't home. Because of the three-day restriction on entering 1105 Mass Ave, I couldn't even get back into the apartment to find the phone number for John's hotel in Singapore.

He was puzzled when no one answered his phone call from Japan. When he reached Singapore and called again, without success, his puzzlement changed to mild consternation. John was a little worried about Katie and me, but not much—he was pretty sure that if there had been some sort of disaster, he would have heard about it. His chief concern was more immediate. I had promised to leave a message at his hotel, relaying some information from a co-worker. The information was a crucial part of a presentation John was scheduled to give to his Asian client shortly after arriving in Singapore. He called again before he went to bed. Still no answer. After three hours of sleep, he tried one more time. Nothing.

This was becoming downright upsetting. John was woozy from fatigue, had a terrible crick in his neck, and could feel another cold coming on. He wasn't in any shape to fake a brilliant performance. The client meeting was due to begin in thirty minutes, and he desperately needed the information I was supposed to have sent hours earlier. John made himself focus on this issue, so that he wouldn't end up drifting into crazy speculations about me and Katie being eaten by a pack of rabid apartment poodles, or attacked by our fat neighbor lady, who just might, now that he thought of it, have revealed an occasional glint of serial-killer psychosis behind her matronly persona. Finally, feeling a trifle on edge, he called his company's corporate headquarters in Cambridge.

John didn't rank high enough at the firm to have his own secretary, but the woman who answered the phone knew him anyway.

"Well, hello, there!" she said. "I saw your wife on the news!"

This was not precisely what John had expected to hear. He just sat there for a second, with his mouth open. Then he collected himself enough to say, "Really?"

"Boy, that was some fire!" said the secretary. "Do you know that ten years ago *to the day*, that very same apartment building burned down? That time, something like forty people were killed! Weird, huh?"

"Burned down?" said John. "My wife? On the news?"

"Boy, did she look bad," said the secretary. "Where were *you*, anyway?"

John jumped to his feet and began pacing around the hotel room, the phone mashed up to his ear. "What happened?" he barked. "Where is she?"

There was a moment of shocked silence before the secretary said, "You mean you don't *know*?"

"Don't know what?" John yelled. "Is Martha all right? Where's my daughter?"

"Uh, well . . ." The secretary stammered, horrified by her faux pas. "I think—I mean, they're fine, at least they looked fine. I mean, not *fine*, fine, but they got out."

"Got *out*?"

"Of the building," she said. And she went on to report everything she had heard on the news about the destruction of Food Shak and the evacuation of the building's inhabitants. John was first horrified, then relieved by the story. When she said that there had been no fatalities, he began to relax.

I'd like to interrupt, at this point, to tell you how I know all this. The easy answer is that John and I have talked about the incident since, in great detail. That is the truth, but it is not the whole truth. The whole truth is that the moment the secretary mentioned my appearance on the news and John began to worry about me, I snapped awake as though something had exploded next to my head. In the thin dawn light of Sibyl and Charles's living room, ten thousand miles away from John, the Seeing Thing was happening, more vividly than it had ever happened before. I could see the hotel room where John was pacing, the view from the window, the remnants of his room-service snack (coffee and a selection of tropical fruit, of which he had eaten everything but the mango).

I could also feel the panic rising in John's chest, then slowly ebbing as his conversation with the secretary continued. I didn't know exactly what he was saying and thinking—the images were visual and emotional—but the *feeling* came through so sharply that my heart began to hammer along with John's. Much later, after lengthy discussion and comparing of notes, John and I came to believe that the Seeing Thing worked best when not only I was thinking of John but he was thinking of me as well. This was also the first time John himself would begin to feel it happening. He didn't see anything, but he had a sudden impression that I was in the room. On my side of the planet, I rubbed my eyes and told myself I was probably dreaming. On his side, John found himself looking around, expecting me to walk out of the hotel bathroom.

"Do you want me to find her for you?" the secretary asked John. She could tell she had scared him, and her voice was apologetic.

"What?" said John. He had been distracted by the sense of my presence, to the point where he hardly remembered the conversation he was having.

"I could do a little detective work," said the secretary. "Try to locate your wife."

John began to say no thanks but stopped. "Actually," he said, "that would be very kind of you. Would you mind?"

"Of course not," she said. "I'll get right on it and call you back."

"Thank you," said John.

They hung up.

That telephone conversation was a watershed for John. For one thing, it was the first time he had ever felt desperate enough to allow his personal life to bleed over into his business persona. Under ordinary circumstances, he would never have mentioned his family to anyone at the office, much less *asked for help,* God save us, on a personal matter. It was also the first time he had completely lost focus on his work, so much that he'd forgotten the original reason for his call. He never even asked the secretary for the information he needed to make his dinner meeting go smoothly.

Predictably, the meeting didn't go very well. John had trouble concentrating on the business at hand—a bizarre and unprecedented experience for him. He kept thinking about me and Katie, and the new baby-to-be. He tried to picture the fetus, though this was difficult. I had told him a great deal about it, forcing him to look at pictures in books that showed various stages of human fetal development, but he'd never really paid much attention. He seemed to recall that the fetus was now about the size of a golf ball. Or maybe a golf tee. He couldn't remember. Something to do with golf. Couldn't be a golf cart, or a golf course. Maybe a golf shoe, one of the smaller sizes . . .

The client, the very important Asian client, was asking John a question, and John hadn't heard a word of it. He gaped at the client for a few seconds, trying to see if he'd stored any words in his short-term memory, but in the end he had to ask the man to repeat the question. When John tried to answer, he found that his vocabulary had diminished to about four words, and he had to fill in the blanks with the syllable *uh*. He could almost feel the eyes of his co-workers boring into him, registering disapproval at the level where his skin was thinnest.

Ordinarily, this would have bothered John immensely. He could never tolerate turning in a performance that was less than perfect. No minuses had ever besmirched the monotonous string of A grades on his report cards and transcripts. But that night in Singapore, John wasn't his usual self. His performance was adequate but not stellar.

The really frightening thing was, *he didn't care.*

It is difficult for a normal, mentally healthy person to understand the enormity of this fact. Most of us humans have long since accepted that a good deal of the work we do is mediocre. But not John. Not only did he come from a long line of obsessive workaholics but he lived in a culture where lovers sign their letters to each other with phrases like "Wishing you a productive summer." Emotionalism and sentiment have no place at Harvard, except as topics of discussion in courses like Nineteenth-Century British Novels or Abnormal Psychology.

As John sat in that Southeast Asian restaurant, paying only dim attention to the conversation, something began to shift inside him. It made him think of the glaciers melting away at the end of the Ice Age: the way he saw the world seemed to be cracking, retreating, dissolving.

These peculiar sensations were both troubling and fascinating. They did not disappear after the dinner meeting. In fact, as he lay in bed that night, he could feel them slowly intensifying. They made John so restless that he finally got up and went for a walk through downtown Singapore. The heavy rain-forest air hung around him, so thick that he wanted to push it aside with his hands, and the lights of the city shone on empty storefronts and the occasional skittering beetle.

I can remember that walk of John's, even though I was picking Katie up at the day-care center, as far away from John as I could be without leaving the planet. I know, because I was with him.

⌐ Of course, I also now know where the massive, tectonic shifts in John's worldview would eventually take him—and me. Adam's arrival transformed our relationship to work more dramatically than any other area of our lives. It is amazing to live with someone who genuinely couldn't care less about Getting Ahead, someone who is absolutely committed to finding joy in the present moment. The belief John and I shared before Adam came along—that rigidly disciplined, distasteful work was the one and only path to a good life—now seems both horrible and downright silly, like believing that we could make it rain by performing human sacrifices. Adam's birth convinced us that fate was quite capable of crushing our best-laid plans like so many dead beetles. In the face of such uncertainty, the only things that seem to us worth doing are the ones that allow us to experience the strange and eventful journey of life in its full richness.

Whenever John and I begin to forget this, our son is there to help us remember. This happens often. For example, there was the Testing

Incident, which occurred shortly after we moved to Arizona. Adam was six at the time. We had spent his baby years in Utah, while I finished my dissertation and John and I taught at the university where both our fathers had worked. Our families, our hometown, and our jobs had offered us the sense of security that comes with familiar things, something we sorely needed after the stressful period of Adam's gestation. By 1993, however, both John and I were beginning to feel confined by our jobs. So one fine day, we both quit. Just up and did it. We didn't have any other source of income waiting for us, but that didn't matter. We'd grown so used to having Bunraku puppeteers all over the place that we were fairly sure they would take care of petty details like money.

Sure enough, after a period of uncertainty and wavering faith that seems brief (though only in retrospect), John was recruited by a business school in Arizona. He had had other job offers, but none of them sounded appetizing to him. In fact, John had turned down the initial offer from the business school as well. It turned out to be a great, though unconscious, negotiating tactic. The school kept coming back to him with revised contracts until they'd structured a job so exactly aligned with John's interests that he actually preferred it to doing nothing. I had decided that I wanted to write books, so I wasn't tied to any geographic location. We moved our family south for John's new job and took to our new environment like hogs to slop.

The only serious difficulty I encountered during our relocation was enrolling Adam in elementary school. I'd heard from other parents of children with Down syndrome that school systems are not always eager to integrate "different" students, and this turned out to be true. The kid had to pass more tests before he was allowed to enter first grade than if he'd applied to be a Green Beret. Every day, after his sisters went to school, he gamely put on his suit and tie and readied himself for another testing session. Hour after hour, we sat in tiny, airless rooms while Special Educators of various stripes put him through a barrage of incredibly boring procedures: IQ tests, vocabulary tests, digital dexterity tests, ear tests, eye tests. At the end of every test Adam was given a small reward, like a can of Sprite, and allowed to go out and play on the swing set.

This was all very well for a while, but eventually Adam got frustrated. This was not the way he remembered school. Where were the other kids? The crayons? The blackboards? I tried to explain what was happening, but the truth was that I didn't know much more than he did about the testing requirements, or the date when he would finally be allowed to go to a regular classroom. We were both getting a little depressed.

And then Adam did something brilliant.

That morning, as usual, Adam and I dropped Lizzie off at her Montessori school and put Katie on the bus headed for third grade. As we pulled up at a stoplight, another yellow school bus stopped beside us.

"Ook, Mom!" said Adam, pointing, "Tatie's bus!"

"No," I said. "That's not Katie's bus. That bus is number five-seven. Katie's is five-nine."

"Five-nine?" Adam repeated. He has this way of asking for more information by repeating what you've just said to him, in a tone that indicates astonished fascination. It's as though you've just explained to him that time is not linear, and he can see the logic of it, but it's so amazing he can't quite quell his astonishment.

"Five-nine," he said again, pondering it. "Tatie's bus is five-nine."

Half an hour later we were sitting in yet another tiny room, watching another special education evaluator (I'll call him Mr. Larvalform) prepare his testing materials. They were pretty simple. The first thing Larvalform pulled out was a stack of cards, each of which had pictures of four objects on it. He held the first card up where Adam could see it.

"I'm just going to ask him to pick out certain objects," Larvalform told me.

"Right." I nodded, feeling my pulse speed up a little. I have had mild testing anxiety on my own behalf from time to time, but if you're a parent you know that this is nothing compared with the anxiety you feel when your kid's future is the one on the line. I couldn't stop fidgeting until Mr. Larvalform asked the first question. Then I relaxed. He was playing right to Adam's strength.

"Adam," he said, "can you point to the *bus*?"

I allowed myself a smile. There it was, in the upper-left-hand quadrant of the card: a yellow school bus. One of Adam's very favorite things.

And yet, he hesitated. He peered at the card as though it were an ancient and inscrutable sheaf of runes he'd dug out of the ground. His well-scrubbed brow furrowed, and he put one finger to his lip in fierce concentration.

"Adam, honey," I said, feeling myself start to sweat, "Adam, point to the bus."

Mr. Larvalform shook his head at me, reminding me to stay out of it. I gave him a little ingratiating smile. "He knows this," I said.

Very slowly, Adam extended his finger and pointed to a picture of a rake.

"No, Adam," said Mr. Larvalform, firmly. "Point to the *bus*."

Adam chewed his lip, eyes completely blank. Then he pointed to an apple.

"No, no!" I burst out in dismay. "Adam, come on, you *know* this." I turned to Mr. Larvalform. "He really does," I said. "He knows it."

Larvalform arched an eyebrow. Meanwhile, Adam appeared to be lapsing into a vegetative state. His head listed to one side, his mouth dropped open, his tongue lolled out, and his eyes crossed. He looked as though he couldn't win a battle of wits with a landed carp.

"Adam," I whispered, as though Mr. Larvalform wouldn't be able to hear me in the five-by-five-foot room. "You little skunk, what are you *doing*?"

He slumped down in his chair like a blob of mud.

"Okay, then," said Mr. Larvalform crisply. He flipped over the card with the bus on it, made a mark on his evaluation sheet, and held up the next card.

"Adam," he said, "can you point to the *dog*?"

There was the dog, plain as day. Adam could *draw* one almost that well. Nevertheless, he raised one lethargic finger and brought it down again on the picture of a feather. It was then that I figured out what was going on.

"Adam!" I said, shocked. "You're *faking* it! Adam, stop it! Stop it right now!"

His eyes slid over toward me in dim recognition. He started to drool.

"Mrs. Beck," said Mr. Larvalform coldly. "Perhaps you'd prefer to wait in the hall?"

"Listen!" I was desperate. "He knows 'bus'! He knows 'dog'! He's acting dumb because he knows that as soon as he maxes out, you'll let him go play on the swing set!"

I was right. Adam had figured out how all placement tests work: the questions start out easy and get harder and harder, until the person being tested isn't able to answer any more. Adam was sick of being tested, he wanted to get out, and he knew exactly how to do it. As I realized this, my son's eyes met mine, uncrossed for an instant, and revealed a brief flash of humor.

"Mrs. Beck," said Larvalform firmly, "I know it's hard to accept, but we need to be realistic about your son's abilities."

"I *am* being realistic!" I said. "I'm telling you, Mr. Larvalform, he's playing you like a piano—he just wants his Sprite!"

This time Adam grinned at me, his eyes sparkling merrily. But by the time Larvalform looked back at him, the lights had gone out again. He half-lay in his chair, staring at his own nose as though it were the only thing in the universe he could even try to understand.

Eventually, I did get the examiner to write my interpretation of that test down on his records. I caught a glance of it later on. It said, "Subject unable to answer Level One vocabulary. Mother claims subject is *'faking it.'*" This made me feel like Dogberry in *Much Ado About Nothing*—you know, the guy who says, "But masters, remember that I am an ass; though it be not written down, yet forget not that I am an ass." I can still picture the school board sitting with that document, sadly shaking their heads over my inability to come to terms with my child's limitations.

Adam had a great time on the swings.

In the long run, he was probably saved from institutionalization by a speech therapist who had a three-year-old son with Down syndrome. She knew perfectly well that Adam was capable of gaming the system.

She saw through his diversionary tactics and placed him in a class where he immediately began to thrive.

⮞ My own way of thinking, living, and working received yet another gentle course correction that day in Mr. Larvalform's tiny office. After spending the first decades of my own life in a desperate attempt to pass every arbitrary test placed before me by the educational system and the rest of society, I have to be constantly reminded that the end goal of all this striving is to live joyfully, and that there are often more direct ways of achieving this than conforming to rigid standards set by social custom.

Strangely enough, this philosophy has actually *become* my career, or at least a good part of it. If you'd told me, ten years ago, that I would one day completely surrender my rigid efforts to conform with "normal" work standards, I would have laughed in your face and then run for the door, like Scrooge fleeing the Ghost of Christmas Yet to Come. Living life as a pursuit of joy would have struck me as lunacy, if not blasphemy. But after a few years of living with Adam, I developed so much confidence in this idea that I became a career counselor. A rather unorthodox career counselor, to be sure. I'm always surprised by the way my clients react to the suggestion that they structure their lives around richness of experience, rather than security. These are educated people, I think to myself. During their many years of training, hasn't anyone ever told them that life is pretty much a crapshoot but one full of unexpected wonders? Hasn't anyone given them permission to live for their hearts' desires?

Then I remember that despite all *my* years of education and training, I have learned most of what I know about living joyfully from one person, and he is not on any faculty. They barely let him into the first grade. Since that night in Singapore when both John and I began to experience the slow warming of our personal Ice Age, we have increasingly taken our retarded son as our own counselor. People pay me good money to pass along to them what Adam teaches me for free. Luckily, I'm pretty sure he will never demand a percentage of the take. It scares me to think how much I owe him.

14

⬝ One of the cruelest things about Harvard is the scheduling of its fall semesters. I don't know who came up with it, but I picture a group of seventeenth-century Puritans sitting around in hair shirts, brainstorming about how they could take as much joy out of the holiday season as possible. Most colleges wrap up the fall semester in time for the holiday season, allowing students to visit family and friends in a state of welcome relaxation before returning for the spring semester. Harvard, by contrast, lets its students go for the holidays with the fall semester still unfinished. Students return to the campus in the coldest, darkest part of the year, facing two more weeks of classwork. They then enter two weeks of "dead" time, during which no classes meet and everyone writes term papers. In my undergraduate years, when people had typewriters rather than computers, you could hear the frantic tap-tap-tap-tap from all directions, around the clock, all the way through Dead Days. Occasionally, the typewriters would be drowned out by the sound of someone screaming out of a dorm window, begging for release like a prisoner in a dungeon. The Dead Days were followed by two weeks of exams, which swiftly destroyed any lingering wisps of mental health that remained among the student body.

This schedule means that just about every Harvard student goes home for the holidays with suitcases full of books and assignments, and firm intentions of catching up in every class before returning to the campus. Of course, no one—or at any rate, no one I could ever really like—actually carries through on this. But the blight of obligation, the pressure to excel, and the fear of failure manage to poison almost everyone's seasonal cheer. You can practically feel John Harvard and the rest of those Puritan forefathers looking down with grim approval on the frigid campus.

As 1987 drew to a close, even after years of experience had taught us how futile it was, John and I packed more work into our vacation bags than ever before. This time, we told each other, we were really going to stay focused. In between visiting our respective families, reconnecting with old friends, and playing Santa for Katie, we were going to Get a Lot Done. We had to. The holiday pressure I had felt during my undergraduate career was nothing compared with graduate school's. This year, I knew that I'd spend exam period grading the papers of the students from my Caribbean Society section rather than studying for my own exams. To make time for this, I planned to have my term papers written well ahead of time. John, of course, would be going back to Singapore as soon as the winter break was over, and absolutely had to finish his Harvard assignments before then. Our carry-on bags were so heavy with books that when I tried to pick mine up I staggered into the wall. I think I actually did read one of those books during winter break—well, maybe just a chapter from one of them. All right, so I didn't exactly *read* it. It was more a kind of skimming behavior. So sue me.

The thing I always failed to calculate into my holiday schedule was the emotional toll and time involved in trying to meet holiday expectations for both my family and John's. Since we had grown up in the same hometown, going home for the holidays usually meant that we were constantly torn between our families' conflicting cultures and traditions. You wouldn't think they'd be all that different, two Utah families descended from similar troops of pioneers, both headed by university professors. Our fathers got their Ph.D.'s from Berkeley in the same year. One of the reasons I married John was that I'd read statistics indicating that the more similar two people's backgrounds are, the more likely it is that they will have a happy and long-lasting marriage. I decided this meant that the fact that John and I were delivered by the same obstetrician was a good thing. (Of course, if John had been from Zimbabwe, I would have found some rationale for marrying him anyway. Those of us who are trained in the social sciences know how to find the data to support whatever we want to be true.) Anyway, despite the similarities in our backgrounds, Christmas was always a festive time to figure out how different my family and John's really were.

The year I was expecting Adam, John's parents were wintering in Arizona. This made our vacation slightly less stressful than in other years, when we would stay with them in the house where John grew up. Everything in that house looked perfect, from the crystal chandelier in the dining room to the hardwood closets in the guest bedroom. There was not a mote of dust on the premises, not a crack in the paint, not a shingle on the roof out of place. Everyone who went into the house, and everything done in it, looked perfect as well. It was an unspoken but clearly understood entrance requirement. My mother-in-law, Faye, cooked well-balanced and delicious meals three times a day, and spent most of the rest of her time cleaning. John's father, Jay (yes, Faye and Jay), was just as attentive to the exterior of the house as his wife was to the interior. They were as refined and gracious as their estate, both small and well groomed and white haired. They reigned over their lovely, immaculate home like Mr. and Mrs. Santa.

As much as I enjoyed and admired my in-laws, their style of thinking and talking was difficult for me to master—particularly when I was pregnant. For one thing, Beck women do not allow themselves to show weakness, much less illness. They just keep cooking and cleaning, stopping occasionally for Polite Conversation. During the Christmas season of 1987, the only activities that sounded even remotely pleasant to me were lying absolutely still and moaning. In her gracious way, my mother-in-law made it very clear to me that she had experienced morning sickness many times but that she had always mastered it by "getting up and getting moving." By this she meant cooking and cleaning, activities that were alien to my nature at the best of times and utterly intolerable when I was in a family way. For the first hour or two after we reached my in-laws' rented condo in Phoenix, I tried to act appropriately Beck-like. But the first time I walked into the kitchen, the central control headquarters for all true Beck women, I threw up so violently that I was positive my head would come off. After that, I gave up on "getting moving." I had to struggle just to meet the barest minimum social requirements by participating in the Polite Conversation.

In Japanese there are two words for "thing": *koto* and *mono. Koto* means an intangible thing, like a concept or behavior or idea. *Mono* means something physical, an object you could hold in your hand. I mean no disrespect when I say that John's clan are *mono* people. The hours and hours and hours of Polite Conversation they engage in whenever they get together center almost entirely on physical objects. They can discuss the maintenance of the flowers in their yard or the recipe for meat loaf for thirty minutes at a stretch, never once letting their attention lag. Whenever they go out to eat, the entire conversation is likely to focus on any changes in the decor or personnel of the restaurant since the last time they were there. The most exotic and highly favored topic for Polite Conversation, however, is airplane travel. When we stayed with the Becks in 1987, with John in the midst of his round-the-world adventures, the conversation rarely strayed from this subject.

"So," my father-in-law asked John, as we sat in the condo's perfect living room, watching a perfect fire crackling in the perfect fireplace, "what airline do you usually travel?"

John paused for three or four seconds before answering. His parents' pace of speech was about one-tenth the Boston norm, and John fell easily into it.

"Singapore Airlines," he said at last.

"Oh," Jay responded, after some thought. "Singapore Airlines."

"Yes," John agreed slowly. "Singapore Airlines."

There was a long silence as everyone took this in. Then my mother-in-law asked, "How's the food on Singapore Airlines?" (The fact that food is served on airplanes apparently created a space for Beck women to enter conversations on the subject.)

"Not bad," John said. "It's good food. I go business class."

"Business class." Jay shook his head. "Amazing."

At this, John and both his parents suddenly emitted a pleasant chuckling sound. No one ever laughed out loud during a Beck conversation, but there was always an enormous amount of pleasant chuckling. I could never tell when it was going to happen, but the Becks all seemed to know when to do it, and they appeared very bonded by the exercise.

"I remember once," Jay continued after a minute or so, "I flew on Singapore Airlines. Let's see, that must have been in about . . . oh, I'd say about 1979 or so." He stopped to think for a minute. "Or maybe it was 1980." More thinking. "No, I think it was 1979. Yes, 1979. Anyway, I'll always remember that stewardess. She had on a red dress."

"No," Faye put in, "it was a blue dress."

"Was it?" Jay's eyebrows lifted in surprise.

"Yes, it was blue. A blue dress."

"Oh. I thought it was red."

More pleasant chuckling all around.

"Yes, it was blue," Faye repeated when the chuckling was over.

"Well, I guess you're right," my father-in-law said. "A blue dress. Anyway, they gave us fish for dinner."

"Ah." John nodded appreciatively. "Fish."

"Yes," Faye put in. "Fish."

Jay: And it was pretty good.

Faye: Did you think so?

Jay: Mine was.

Faye: I thought it was a little dry.

Jay: Oh, really?

Faye: Yes. Mine was.

Jay: Huh! Well, mine was pretty good.

Long before this point, I had begun pinching myself violently to keep from lapsing into a coma. Despite their sincere affection and the comfort of familiar communication patterns, a Polite Conversation at the Becks' affected me like chloroform. I looked over at John for support and comfort, but he was sitting there with this goony little-boy smile on his face, like a duck that had been brought back to its pond after a long hike through the desert.

Of course, I wanted very much for John's family to like me, and he was very anxious for me to make the right impression, so sometimes I'd try to participate in the Polite Conversation. It didn't come naturally to me, but I'd do my best to pitch in with a comment or two. It would go something like this:

Faye: Well, I guess I'll go over to Jolyn's tomorrow and get my hair done.

Jay: Jolyn? I thought that woman named Bernice did your hair.

Faye: No, she moved. Now I go to Jolyn's.

Jay: Huh! Jolyn's!

Faye: I didn't like Bernice much anyway. She made my hair look terrible.

Everyone Except Martha: Chuckle chuckle chuckle.

John: So, you'll be going over to Jolyn's. Does she do a good job?

Faye: Oh, a pretty good job. I like the way she combs it out.

Jay: Huh! Well, it looks good.

John: Yeah, Mom, it looks great.

Faye: Yes, Jolyn does a pretty good job.

Martha: You know, humans are the only species of primate that don't do much mutual grooming. I think that's why women talk so much to their hairdressers. Being groomed sort of triggers the old social-bonding instinct. Don't you think that's likely?

At this, all the Becks would stare at me in mute, unanimous horror for about thirty seconds, after which they would begin to talk about airplanes. Later, when we had retired to the guest bedroom, John would throw a minor fit because I had been so rude, and I would try to hit him with the cardboard tube from a festive roll of holiday gift wrap, and we would go to sleep in icy silence.

ᔆ   The visit to my family was—er—somewhat different. The house I grew up in was not on the slopes of the Wasatch mountains, where the Becks and all the other respectable folks in town had their homes. Our house was down on the valley floor, which was inhabited mainly by college students and poor white trash. My family intersected with both these groups, without really being part of either. My father was a well-respected professor, a popular speaker not only at the university but also in the community at large. That made my family part of the college crowd. However, our modest family income, the number of children in the family (eight), and above all, the condition of our house, kept us in the poor-white-trash range, socially speaking.

That house was the bane of my existence. I still have nightmares about it. It was a small brick structure that my parents, in some fit of pathological creativity, had painted swimming-pool blue. The house was this color when I was born and had never been repainted by the time I left for college. Small, crackling strips of swimming-pool-blue paint kept flaking off the house and dropping to the ground around it, giving lead poisoning to the many stray cats who lived in our garage. The garage itself was overflowing with junk, far too much of it to leave room for a car. That was all right, though, because no amount of weathering could have made the car look worse. It was a little yellow Datsun, so old and battered that the doors flew open every time the car went around a curve. My parents had solved this problem by placing loops of twine around the headrests of the seats, then hooking the twine around the little lock knobs on the doors.

The car spent its time next to a yard that was completely covered with dead leaves. My father believed that they would act as mulch for the grass. Every autumn, he not only left the leaves that fell directly onto our lawn but raked leaves off the street and sidewalk onto the yard, bizarrely confident that the next spring grass would burst through the leaves in emerald splendor. In every season, the yard looked sort of like a compost heap, only drier.

The inside of the house was even worse than the outside. Much worse. When I was growing up, my many older siblings warned me not to let anyone near our house, and to throw myself in front of a speeding car rather than let anyone actually go inside. They told me that if any of our acquaintances ever realized how we lived, we would all become instant pariahs at school. They were probably right.

To begin with, my parents' mysterious color preferences showed up in every room. The living room, for example, had walls and carpet of a pale mint-green hue (although the carpet was so dirty it was hard to tell the color). Sitting near the center of the living room was an easy chair made of hunter-orange polyester, which my parents had purchased with

Gold Strike Stamps, thinking it would create a nice contrast with the walls. Contrast, yes. Nice, no.

Granted, it was hard to really see the color scheme in the house, because every horizontal surface was covered with Stuff. I don't even know what the Stuff was. I'm sure—you'll think I'm exaggerating, but I am not—that some of my elementary school homework was still lodged amid the Stuff when John and I visited my ancestral lodge in December of 1987. The Stuff reached heights of eighteen inches or more on the seats of chairs, the tops of tables and shelves, and strategic parts of the floor. I still have a habit of sitting down on things without even noticing them, a skill my whole family had to master if we wanted to sit down at all. When we were growing up, my siblings and I would occasionally launch a desperate attempt to clean the house, but it never got very far. There were too many of us in too small a space, and the place was way too far gone for cleaning long before my time.

Couched as we were in the middle of so much unattractive Stuff, my siblings and I had grown up with a forced obliviousness to *mono,* to tangible objects. Every trace of self-esteem and family pride we managed to dredge up had to do with *koto*—ideas, theories, concepts. All of this was based on my father's legendary intellectual brilliance. He was a bona fide genius, who did research in upwards of twenty languages and held dozens of book-length works of literature and philosophy in his memory. Everyone in town had heard of him, and most recognized him on sight. My teachers often asked me what it was like to be raised by the smartest man in the community. Despite our unkempt appearance and lack of social graces, my father's much-lauded intelligence gave us all a certain dignity, and high status among our peers.

Brains were everything in my family. Some of the few visitors allowed into our house when I was little were college students studying psychology and child development, who had been given assignments that necessitated interacting with actual children. My siblings and I were pretty much the only children in the neighborhood. As a result, we were frequently subjected to various types of experimentation, involving everything from simple observation to testing our IQs. My parents were always especially happy to let them measure our IQs.

I remember taking one IQ test with my father in the room, looking on. I was three or four, and the psychology student had me sit on the floor while she gave me a number of tests designed to measure memory and analytical ability. She also tested my vocabulary. My father was standing behind her, and I could see from the expression on his face that he was deeply invested in the outcome of the tests. At one point the researcher asked me the question "Do dogs manufacture?"

I was unsure of the correct response. I knew that *manufacture* meant to make something, and while I had never heard anyone say that dogs manufactured anything, I was sure of two things they made: puppies and poop.

"Yes," I said uncertainly, hoping she wouldn't ask me any specific questions about the poop.

My father reacted as though he'd been stung by a bee. He had kept quiet up to that point, as the student researcher had requested, but this was too much for him.

"No, no, no, no, *no!*" he said, bouncing up onto the balls of his feet as he did when he got excited. "Dogs don't manufacture! Think of the Latin roots—*manu* means 'hand,' *facture* means 'make.' To make with the hands. Dogs don't even *have* hands, you idiot!"

Idiot was a popular word in my house. We all used it frequently. It referred to anyone who wasn't as smart as my father, and it protected us against the humiliation that might have been imposed upon us by our hand-me-down clothes and our horrible house. Anyone who made fun of us, or lived in a nicer place, or wore expensive clothes was manifestly an idiot, and therefore beneath contempt. Given this strategy for propping up our self-esteem, it is little wonder that my siblings and I were very concerned about the results of our IQ tests.

My father was actually in the first wave of American children to take intelligence quotient tests when they were developed. After the results of those first tests came back, the principal of my father's elementary school called him in and told him, "Hugh, if you were to go to sleep right now, and stay asleep for nine years, and your classmates kept studying that whole time, you would still be ahead of them when you woke up."

This was the type of story that got me and mine through the shame of growing up in squalor. It was the kind of story we retold every year when we gathered together amid the piles of Stuff to celebrate the holidays. We retold it at top volume, all eight siblings shouting to get a word in edgewise. This was the way we always talked when you got a group of us together. The conversation ripped along at breakneck speed and numbing volume, filled with stiletto humor, double entendres, puns, and allusions. Anyone who couldn't keep up, or who said something stupid, would be turned upon and verbally mauled for a few minutes, until someone else did something equally "idiotic," and the focus of ridicule would shift.

Occasionally, especially at celebratory times, the whole gang of us would launch into a spontaneous mental game. For example, my mother used to send me to our back porch (a room containing no furniture but a simply incredible mass of Stuff) to get flour for holiday cakes or pies. I often returned to the kitchen, cringing with disgust, to announce that the flour was full of worms. No matter how sick this made me, I knew it wouldn't bother my mother. She always just sifted the worms out, saying that even if she missed a few and they got into the food, they would simply be an excellent source of protein. Just as we were all beginning to feel thoroughly downtrodden, my father would save the day. "Everyone come up with a literary reference about worms!" he would shout.

There would be a sudden silence as everyone thought furiously, trying to come up with the first, the best, the most worm references. Then someone would shout, *"Moby-Dick!* Maggots in the ship's biscuits!"

"Thomas Aquinas! *Wurms!"* someone else would yell. And the literary contest would be off and running. It was here, among my flesh and blood, that my alter ego, Fang, had first learned the fine art of intellectual competition. My family might be worm eaters, but by damn, we were smart.

As you can imagine, bringing John into this group was like throwing a purebred, rigidly trained champion show dog into a pack of junkyard mutts. John had learned witty repartee in his club at Harvard, but the pace, intensity, and decibel level of my family's banter was hard to match. I knew John could hold his own with my family, and I kept waiting for him to leap into the verbal fray, but he never did. It felt completely alien to him. The chaos of voices and the abundance of Stuff made him feel dazed and swamped, like a computer with too much data being dumped into the hard drive. He would respond to this in the only way permissible in his family system: his eyes would glaze over, and he would sit there emitting the pleasant chuckling noise until he fell abruptly, inexplicably, profoundly asleep. Later, when we had retired for the night, I would throw my own fit at his unwillingness to even *try* to fit in with my family, and he would go into a huffy silence, and we would, once again, end the day as enemies.

Christmas vacations had been this way ever since John and I were married. This is one reason it was so absurd of us to pack dozens of academic books in our luggage. Surrounded by the masses of social pressure from our families of origin, and preoccupied by the battles that inevitably ensued between us after we interacted with them, John and I both allowed Harvard to fade into the furthest reaches of our conscious minds. Instead, our families' priorities came roaring back from childhood; John remembered once again how absolutely essential it was to look perfect at all times, and I once again set out to prove that I was not an idiot.

Both these impulses would make it very difficult for us to handle the months ahead, but at the time they were actually a welcome distraction. They not only put Harvard in a different perspective but also helped me cope with the nausea that was still my constant companion. The concerns I had developed about the health of my unborn child now seemed ridiculously unfounded. I put them aside, along with the academic books I was supposed to be reading.

John and I knew, as we did every year, that the relaxation would end with a jolt once we returned to school. Back at Harvard, our professors were waiting for our term papers, our students were waiting for their grades. What I did not know was that the obstetrical nurse-practitioner at University Health Services, who had just received the results of my blood tests, was waiting for me to return her increasingly desperate messages. If she couldn't get in touch with me soon, she was afraid it was going to be too late.

15

↷ We had turned off the heat to our apartment when we left for the holiday break, and when we returned, the place was so cold that our breath not only froze but actually drifted toward the floor in tiny crystal clouds. It seemed to me, as I let Katie out of her stroller and turned up the thermostat, that this apartment had always been cold, even in summer. The chill was more psychological than physical. The three sparsely furnished rooms overlooking Harvard Square contained places to study, places to work, places to close our eyes for a few exhausted hours before going back to work again, but not really places to live.

The furnace began to pump warm air soon enough, but I left my coat on while I listened to the messages on the answering machine. I was glad I did. The first message sent an icy shiver through me.

"Martha, this is the nurse-practitioner at University Health Services." The voice sounded urgent, frustrated, almost angry. "I need to get in touch with you immediately—*immediately*—regarding the results from one of the tests you requested. *Please* get in touch with me as soon as possible."

She left the phone number, and I scribbled it on a piece of paper with cold-stiffened fingers. When I looked up, John was standing in the bedroom doorway with Katie in his arms and a look of startled concern on his face.

"What's that about?" he said, nodding toward the answering machine.

I shook my head. "I don't know." But I did know. The gut feeling that something was wrong with the baby had just resurfaced and received an unwelcome validation.

"Probably no big deal," said John, flashing me his deceptively confident smile.

"Right," I said. "No big deal."

"You'd better call her, anyway." John's voice was still casual, but it had an undertone that meant he was as anxious as I was.

The nurse-practitioner answered her phone immediately. I liked this woman very much. She was one of the few medical personnel at University Health Services who actually might have recognized me on the street. While the OB-GYN doctors rushed through the clinic, checking as many pregnant women as possible in the brief time they had to spend there, the nurse-practitioner had (or simply took) the time to really talk to each expectant mother. I'll call her Judy Trenton.

"Hi, Judy," I said when she answered the phone. "This is Martha Beck."

"Martha!" Judy said. "I've been trying to reach you!" Her voice took on the tinge of anger I had heard on the answering machine.

"Look," she went on, "when you request tests and then leave town, you really must give us numbers where you can be reached. You really shouldn't even be leaving—what are we supposed to do when the tests show a problem? You have no idea how much time I've spent trying to track you down."

"I'm sorry," I said unhappily. "When the tests show a problem." Not "if." "When." I could feel my heart speeding up, half of me wanting desperately to know what was wrong, the other half ready to slam the phone down without listening.

"So, is there something wrong?" I managed to keep my voice calm, but my hands were shaking.

Judy's voice went back to its usual crisp-but-warm timbre. "Well, we got an unusual reading on your alpha-fetoprotein levels," she said.

"The AFP?" I remembered that a high AFP indicated spina bifida, a condition in which the unborn baby's spinal cord fails to fuse. I had a sudden, horrible image of a baby born with its back open and its internal organs partially outside the skin.

"How high was the level?" I said.

"It wasn't high," said Judy. "It was actually a bit below normal."

"Below normal?" I repeated. "Well, that's good, isn't it?"

Judy made a noncommittal sound. "It's not necessarily *bad*," she said. "But there is a slight statistical correlation between low levels of AFP and Down syndrome."

I felt an immediate surge of revulsion. "Slight," I said at last. "A *slight* statistical correlation."

"Yes, you shouldn't worry," she said. "We just want to do the test again, to see if we get the same results. Just to be on the safe side."

"How slight?" Now I was the one with tension in my voice. "What's the correlation between this and Down syndrome?"

"It depends," she said.

"What are my odds?" I snapped. Fang was awake now, and she was not in the mood for vagueness.

"Well"—I could hear Judy flipping through papers. "It depends on the actual level, and your age. . . . Okay, here, I've got your file. How old are you?"

"Twenty-five."

We were both silent for a minute. John came back into the bedroom and stood silently, watching my face. I didn't meet his eyes. Then Judy said, "All right, I've got it. Based on this one test—which is only preliminary, of course—your odds of having a Down's baby are one in eight hundred ninety-five."

I almost laughed. "Eight hundred ninety-five?" I said. "*That's* why you were chasing me all over the country?"

"You're right not to worry about it," said Judy. The warmth was back in her voice. "But we would like you to come in to repeat the test today. We just want to be on the safe side."

"Today?" I said, rather taken aback. It usually took me a couple of weeks just to get an appointment.

"You're at eighteen weeks' gestation right now," Judy told me. "We don't have much time."

I was confused. "Time? Time for what?"

"To terminate," she said. "If there's something wrong."

I felt the chill again, despite all that heavy clothing and central heating.

"Oh," I said. "Of course."

I shook my head, irritated at myself for being so worried. I was young, I was healthy, I was from a large family with no genetic defects to speak of. Even my morning sickness, as unpleasant as it was, signaled a healthy pregnancy. I scheduled the blood test.

A few hours later, John walked me over to the clinic. Katie rode in her backpack on his shoulders. A light snow was falling on Harvard Square. Students had returned from the holidays, the many restaurants were back in full operation, and the smell of food drifted on warm eddies through the freezing air. The lights of the storefronts, the snowdrifts on people's hats and collars, the bright pink of Katie's cheeks, all struck me as festive and somehow tinged with nostalgia, as though I were looking back on a time of my life that had already passed. I had a strong sense that a chapter was ending, and another was about to begin. I said nothing about this feeling to John. It was too surreal, I thought, too hard to describe.

"*Natsukashii,*" said John as we passed a French bakery and headed toward the door of University Health Services.

"What?" I looked at him sharply.

"Nothing," he said. But I'd already heard him. *Natsukashii* is a Japanese word that described exactly what I was feeling: a wistful sense of longing, an appreciation for beauty laced with sadness at its transience. I fell back half a step and watched John trudge through the snow, wondering why we both felt as though we were going to a funeral.

It took the nurse all of thirty seconds to poke another hole in my arm and extract enough blood to fill several test tubes. It took a bit longer to bring me around after I stood up too fast and plopped to the floor. All in all, John and Katie spent only ten minutes in the waiting room.

John grinned at me as I waddled out of the elevator. I stood on my toes to kiss Katie, still riding in her backpack. We headed for a soup-and-salad restaurant near the clinic.

"So," said John, when we had stationed Katie in her high chair and ordered lunch, "how was it?"

I shrugged. "They just took more blood. Personally, I think they've got a vampire on the staff and they're storing snacks."

"Did they tell you anything else about the test?" John said. "What exactly is the problem?"

I shook my head. "The nurse who took my blood didn't know anything about it. The best info is what Judy told me—we've got a one in eight hundred and ninety-five shot at a retarded baby."

John smiled. "I can live with those odds."

I tried to smile back, but I couldn't. "I'm still . . ." I wanted to tell John about the worry in my gut. I wanted to tell him that it was more than worry—that it was a certainty. Then I realized all over again how preposterous that was. "I'm still a little scared."

He reached across the table for my hand. "Sure," he said. "That's understandable. But even if there's a problem, we've caught it in time."

"In time?" That phrase again.

"Yeah," said John. "The worst-case scenario is that you might have to have an abortion, and that's a long shot. Everything's going to be fine."

I stared at him. "I might have to have an abortion? *Have to?*"

John opened a package of saltines and gave the crackers to Katie. "Look, Marth, the odds are so slim that—"

"I might *have to have* an abortion?" The chill inside me was gone. Instead I could feel my face flushing hot with anger. "Since when do you decide what I *have to* do with my body?"

John looked surprised. "I never said I was going to decide anything," he protested. "It's just that if the tests show something wrong with the baby, of course we'll abort. We've talked about this."

I closed my eyes, trying to rein in my temper. John was right. We'd discussed abortion in general, once or twice, and both of us thought it was a very good idea to abort fetuses with birth defects. I remembered saying so. But now that I was actually pregnant, now that the abortion in question concerned a baby I could already feel moving inside me, the very idea that anyone could say I "had to" end my pregnancy filled me with an almost primeval rage.

"What we've talked about," I told John in a low, dangerous voice, "is that I am pro-choice. That means *I* decide whether or not I'd abort a baby with a birth defect. You steer clear of this one, John-boy. It is *not* your call!"

John looked at me as though I'd slapped him. The anger in my voice shocked even me.

"I'm . . . I'm sorry," I said. "I shouldn't have—I'm not mad. It's just the hormones."

"Whatever," said John. He regarded me warily as the waitress came back from the kitchen with our lunch.

"It's just not ethically consistent," I told John, as soon as the waitress went away.

He took a bite of his sandwich. "What isn't?"

"Abortion," I said. "I mean, not abortion in general, just *this* kind of abortion. This designer-baby stuff."

"You mean screening for birth defects?" John was giving me his surprised look every couple of seconds. "What in the world is wrong with it? It's better for everyone."

I shook my head. "I'm not so sure of that."

"You used to be," said John.

"I know. I used to be." I rubbed my eyes. I felt terribly confused. "But now . . . look, John, it's not as though we're deciding whether or not to have a baby. We're deciding what *kind* of a baby we're willing to accept. If it's perfect in every way, we keep it. If it doesn't fit the right specifications, whoosh! Out it goes."

John shook his head. "Don't be silly, Marth," he said. "You know that isn't true. We're talking about the difference between a healthy, normal baby and a defective one."

The word *defective* hit me like a hammer. I folded my arms across my growing abdomen as if I could shield the baby from it. I felt irrationally, almost violently protective.

"So what exactly is a 'defective' baby?" I demanded.

"Calm down!" John threw an embarrassed glance around the restaurant.

I lowered my voice. "I mean, I know there are babies born so damaged they can't survive on their own," I said, "but what about the ones that would actually live unless they were aborted? Where do you draw the line? Is a baby with only one hand 'defective'?"

John's eyes widened. "Did they say something about its hands?"

"No, no, no," I said irritably. "But what if they did? What if this baby had a clubfoot or something? Would you tell me I 'had to have' an abortion?"

John was looking more and more confused. "Martha, why are you on this soapbox? What's your point?"

"My point is," I said, "that I'm trying to get you to tell me what you think constitutes a 'defective' baby. What about . . . oh, I don't know, a hyperactive baby? Or an ugly one?"

"They can't test for those things, and—"

"Well, what if they could?" I said. "Medicine can do all kinds of magical tricks these days. Pretty soon we're going to be aborting babies because they have the gene for alcoholism, or homosexuality, or manic-depression."

I grabbed Katie's cheese sandwich from her high chair tray and started chopping it into bite-size pieces with my butter knife. I think I looked a little deranged, because both John and Katie just sat there, eyes wide, watching.

"Did you know that in China they abort a lot of fetuses just because they're female?" I growled. "Is being a girl 'defective' enough for you?"

"I didn't say—" John began, but I cut him off again. Words I had never consciously thought were spilling out of me in a torrent, as though I had been desperate to say them for a long, long time.

"Just exactly how smart does a baby have to be before its parents accept it?" I said. "How good-looking? How healthy? How strong?" I was holding the butter knife in my closed fist, pointing it at John, poking it forward a little with every question. John waited until he was sure I wasn't going to stab him, then reached over and gently took the knife out of my hand.

"Honey," he said firmly. "This is not eugenics. We aren't talking about breeding a race of supermen. We're talking about taking some of the tragedy out of life."

I squinted at him. "And you think that aborting an abnormal fetus does that?"

John nodded. "Yeah. I do."

I shook my head. "You are so damn male," I said. "You guys think that just because a baby isn't born yet, it doesn't exist. Get rid of it before a man ever sees it, and it never even happened. Well, that's bullshit, buddy. Ask any woman who's five months pregnant whether her baby exists or not. Then, just for laughs, consider for once that her viewpoint might actually count for something!"

"Martha!" John said. "Don't swear in front of Katie!"

Katie was mashing a sodden saltine into her mouth. She looked from me to John and back in observant silence.

"My point is," I said, "that if a baby is conceived with a birth defect, that's a tragedy. Not if it's *born* with a birth defect, but if it has a birth defect, period. It doesn't matter whether you abort it or let it live. It's a tragedy either way."

Suddenly, my eyes filled with tears. I knew I was grieving, but I didn't know why. The Bunraku puppeteers seemed to be crowding around me, somber and patient, but relentless. John was aghast. This was not the way Beck women comported themselves, particularly not in public. He didn't know what to do.

"Look, honey, nothing's wrong with our baby," he said. "Our baby is *fine*. And yes, I agree with you that birth defects are a tragedy any way you look at it, but abortion is a way to *deal* with the problem, you know? To limit it. That's all I was saying."

I wiped my eyes with a paper napkin and peered at my husband's weary, frustrated face.

"And you'd still want me to abort this baby if it wasn't normal," I said. "Wouldn't you?"

John pulled in a deep breath and let it out slowly. He looked terribly tired.

"Look," he said. "I know I can't always see things from your perspective, and I'm sorry about that. But the way I see it, if a baby is going to be deformed or something, abortion is a way to keep everyone from suffering—*especially* that baby. It's like shooting a horse that's broken its leg." John's father had been born to a clan of sheepherders, and he was always quick with barnyard analogies.

"A lame horse dies slowly, you know?" said John. "It dies in terrible pain. And it can't run anymore, so it can't enjoy life even if it doesn't die. Horses live to run; that's what they *do*. If a baby is born not being able to do what other people do, I think it's better not to prolong its suffering."

I nodded. The torrent of emotion seemed to be passing. I felt as though a hurricane had swept through me, leaving me hollow and exhausted. I swallowed a mouthful of orange juice and closed my eyes.

"And what is it," I said softly, more to myself than to John, "what is it that people *do*? What do we live to do, the way a horse lives to run?"

I didn't expect an answer, and John didn't give one. He just moved his chair closer to mine and put an arm around my shoulders. "You're awfully tired, aren't you?"

I nodded, trying to hold back another wave of tears.

"Let's get you home," he said, stroking my hair. "You look so pale—how much blood did the vampire nurses take, anyway?"

I managed to smile. "Just enough for their midnight buffet."

John smiled and began to laugh. Then, abruptly, he fell silent. He held very still for a moment. Then he said, "What?"

I opened my eyes. John was looking at me, his brow furrowed.

"I didn't say anything," I told him.

He looked confused. "Then who did? Who said that?"

Now I was the perplexed one. "Who said what?"

John turned his head, looking all around the table. There was no one near us.

"John? Are you okay?"

He shook his head slightly. "I'm . . . yes, I'm fine. It's just jet lag. I guess."

I didn't question him any further. I knew, with the kind of knowledge that comes from your core, what had just happened. The puppeteers were talking to John. I was so sure of this that I didn't even bother to articulate it in my own mind. I didn't know what they had said, or why. I would learn those things later. At the time, I just rested my face against John's chest and closed my eyes again.

John brought his other arm around and folded me to his chest. He was still wearing his bulky down parka. It was like a pillow against my cheek. I could feel his heart beating beneath the coat. For a moment, I let the anxiety in my chest relax, let myself forget everything I had to do that day, let myself feel utterly safe. And then I understood that John was answering my question, even though he didn't know he was. This is it, I thought. This is the part of us that makes our brief, improbable little lives worth living: the ability to reach through our own isolation and find strength, and comfort, and warmth for and in each other. This is what human beings *do*. This is what we live for, the way horses live to run.

16

∾ I just cut Adam's hair. I've been cutting it since he was a baby, and until today I have made unilateral command decisions about styling. His hair is the color and texture of corn silk, and I've always left as much of it on his head as I possibly could. Today, however, Adam and both his sisters (along with John and my friend Karen, who lives with us) got together and decided that he needed a new look. It took them a while to persuade me, but ultimately I gave in to the pressure and cut it the way they wanted me to. Now Adam's hair is short all over, with one stylish lock left a bit longer in the front. It's very dashing. His head looks like a dandelion just before the fluff blows away. No one who's seen Adam since the haircut has been able to resist the temptation to run up and rub it with both hands. The kid is walking around charged with so much static electricity I'm afraid he's going to burst into flame.

I am very relieved to see that Adam's new 'do looks good on him, because it was not easy for me to pick up my handy home clippers and shear almost all the hair off my son. Before I let the family talk me into doing this, I informed them that in ancient China, cutting one's hair was considered an insult to one's mother. This makes sense, if you think about it. You didn't make your own hair. Your parents provided all the raw materials, and your mother was a rent-free production facility. (This argument didn't impress my family, who reminded me that I routinely allow my children to insult me in any number of ways.) We Americans aren't nearly as big on filial piety as the Imperial Chinese, but still, I have never met a mother of any culture who could just whack off her children's hair without a few bittersweet twinges. It's so astonishing to look at a child, an incredibly complex, independent living being, and know that it emerged from your own insides. It seems a pity to throw any of it away.

I know an eighty-year-old woman who is still amazed whenever she watches her own children, even though those children are now grand-parents themselves. "Look!" she still says to herself. "Look—they're *alive!*" The incredulity never wanes entirely. But I think there are few experiences to match the very first time a mother lays eyes on her child. It was one of the things I looked forward to most when I knew I was expecting Adam—one of the things that held me back from an early abortion, and helped me get through even the worst of the physical misery.

I had vivid memories of the first time I saw Katie. At the time I had been in labor for forty hours and was so completely exhausted that I had all but forgotten why I was there. My only thought was to get through the next contraction. The obstetrician, who had stayed with me through the entire process and was almost as tired as I was, delivered Katie's head and then suctioned out her throat while I rested before pushing her body out. There I was, draped in my little hospital napkin-shift, surrounded by medical personnel, dazed with pain and fatigue, and still pretty much pregnant. Then, in the middle of all this hurly-burly, I suddenly heard a small cough.

I was confused. It sounded like a *baby,* of all things! I looked around, wondering who on earth had brought a baby into this sterile, high-stress, professional scenario. This was a hospital, not a nursery! Then I heard the small cough again. This time John said, "Gee, it's . . . uh . . . it's pretty purple."

He was looking at me—specifically, at that portion of me which I had always been warned to keep strictly to myself, and which was now being viewed by more strangers than you could fit in a minivan. It dawned on me slowly. Oh, my God, I thought. That was *my* baby who coughed. *I* brought a baby into this room! A person no one had ever seen before, an actual human being who had never existed until now!

A few seconds later Katie's body emerged, looking very purple indeed. The doctor let John cut the umbilical cord (a privilege from which, I am proud to say, he recovered without psychiatric intervention), and the nurse wiped Katie off and put her on my chest. We lay there, my daughter and I, looking at each other, and I don't know which of us was more astonished. I had been prepared for absolutely everything that was going to happen when I gave birth, and still it took me completely by surprise.

Seeing Adam for the first time was even more surreal. It happened just a few days after my second AFP test, some four months before he was born. The results of the second blood test had come back in the low-normal range, meaning that there was no reason to fear Adam had Down syndrome. However, I had badgered Judy Trenton with so many questions and concerns that she suggested I might want to schedule an amniocentesis, a procedure in which fluid is taken from the uterus and analyzed for fetal abnormality.

"We've got a terrific physician who's studying prenatal diagnosis of birth defects with ultrasound," Judy told me, "and your AFP results would justify the amniocentesis to the insurance company."

"You mean they'll pay for it?" I said. "The whole thing?" Amniocentesis is often offered to women who have their children later in their reproductive years, but since I was still quite young, my insurance coverage didn't include the test.

"I'm pretty sure I can convince them to pick up the tab," said Judy. "And it would give us useful data that could help other pregnant women in the future."

This was great. A way to absolutely protect myself from any degree of uncertainty, to put my mind thoroughly at rest. A test that was in some way altruistic and, more important, free. "Let's do it," I said.

⌐ The ultrasound clinic was space age and luxurious, very different from the stark, utilitarian, metal-and-linoleum look at University Health Services. The whole place was carpeted, and even the walls had a textured fabric covering that made them look soft and pleasant. All that cloth muffled sounds, so that everyone in the waiting room seemed to be whispering. Come to think of it, maybe everyone actually was whispering. The group of people waiting for appointments was very different from those I saw at UHS. For one thing, there were as many men as women—almost everyone there seemed to have come in a couple.

For another thing, no one was smiling. There was none of the light-hearted banter you often see between expectant parents. As I signed my-self in and John and I found seats, I realized that all of these women were here not for ordinary prenatal treatment but for the express pur-pose of finding out whether something was drastically wrong with the babies they carried.

After a long wait in that hushed anteroom, John and I were ushered into a small examination area. There were several complicated, impres-sive-looking machines next to the table where I was supposed to lie down. One of them had a little screen, like a television, mounted above a keyboard and attached to a device that looked like a miniature metal detector. As I changed into the paper nerd suit that is the preferred fash-ion statement for all medical environments, John began poking around the device.

"This must be the ultrasound thing," he said, picking up the metal detector. It had a plastic handle, which was attached to a flat metal disk. John held the disk to his ear, then rubbed it along his forearm.

"Put that down," I said. "You're going to break it."

"No, I'm not." He poked at the buttons on the keyboard.

"John!"

"I'm just seeing how it works." John, like many men, has never out-grown his two-year-old curiosity about shiny toys. "Look," he said. "I think this is how you turn it on." He pressed another button. Nothing happened.

"John, cut it out! It looks fragile!"

"Oh, not really," said a voice from the doorway. John jumped a little and stuffed the metal-detector paddle back into its position on the ma-chine. I arched an eyebrow at him.

"Hi, I'm Susan." A tall woman in a spotless, pale blue uniform came into the room and extended her hand to John. He shook it guiltily, cast-ing a nervous glance at the ultrasound machine. "And you must be Martha." Susan smiled as she held out her hand to me. "Nice to meet you both."

We said that it was nice to meet her, too.

"I'm the technical assistant for the amnio," said Susan. "I'll be doing an initial ultrasound exam before the doctor gets here. She'll do the actual amniocentesis."

I nodded, trying not to look too eager. The ultrasound was the real reason I had asked for this procedure. Whenever I was pregnant, I had recurring dreams about being able to see the baby through the tissues of my abdomen, to check on it and note how it was growing. The chance to see my unborn baby with the help of an ultrasound machine was literally a dream come true.

Susan turned off the lights. The room was warm and close and somehow intimate in the dark. I felt as though I had gone back to the womb myself.

"Martha, would you mind lying back on the table? Just get comfortable." Susan's voice sounded louder when I couldn't see her.

I eased myself onto my back, startled, as I always was, by the way my abdomen stood up in a solid lump. Susan looked like a bluish ghost floating through the room. She took something that looked like a plastic mustard bottle from a shelf beneath the screen. Then she moved my nerd suit aside to expose my midsection.

"This may be a little chilly," she warned, squeezing the bottle onto my abdomen. The clear gel that emerged was, indeed, very cool. I shivered.

"Sorry about that," Susan said, and I could see the white flash of her teeth in the darkness as she smiled. "The gel helps conduct the ultrasound through your skin."

She picked up the little metal-detector paddle. "This is the transducer," she said. "It sends sound waves through your tissues and creates an image based on the way the waves bounce back."

"Like radar?" John said.

"Something like that."

This was all old news to me. I had read up on ultrasound at some length. The technique is used for performing amniocentesis because a needle has to be inserted into the uterus, and doctors want to avoid poking the fetus with it. I had read that the images on the ultrasound screen would be vague and fuzzy, and that only a trained technician or physician would be able to "read" them.

Susan pulled the machine with the TV screen closer to the examination table. Then she turned to John. "This is the power button," she said. "Would you like to turn it on?" Her smile flashed again.

"You go ahead," said John sheepishly. Susan laughed as she turned on the ultrasound machine and the screen lit up. It showed only gray static.

"This is one of the highest-definition ultrasound machines in the world," Susan told us. "You may have heard that we are developing a diagnostic test for Down syndrome that uses only ultrasound. It's quicker and a lot less invasive than amniocentesis, but it does require state-of-the-art equipment."

She manipulated some of the buttons on the keyboard, and the static on the screen changed to show a triangle of light, like a slice of pie.

"This shouldn't hurt at all," Susan told me as she put the head of the transducer on my abdomen. I wasn't worried, but I could feel my heart thumping hard with excitement. John reached out to take one of my hands. Both of us were staring at the screen.

"Okay," said Susan. "There's the back." She slid the transducer around on my belly, trying to get a better angle. "See that? That's a leg."

"Oh, right," I said. On the screen, an out-of-focus white cylinder moved in the pie slice of light.

"There's the head." Susan pointed to a blob at the bottom of the screen. "Let's have a look at the bone structure."

She punched a few buttons, and the image on the screen sprang into recognizable shapes: a tiny rib cage, the complicated ridge of a spine, a pelvis.

"Wow!" whispered John. "Look, honey, we're having a skeleton! Let's name it Igor."

I didn't answer. I was utterly captivated by the image on the screen. One of the small legs, its joints still formed of delicate-looking cartilage rather than bone, kicked lazily across the screen. An arm reached out, one small hand touching a foot, feeling it. The baby moved like a diver in deep water.

"Skeletal structure looks good," said Susan. "Now I'm going to have a look at the organs. This machine gives us more capacity to look at soft tissues than any other technology around."

She punched more buttons, and the image went fuzzy again. Then, as Susan readjusted the transducer on my belly, the screen divided into a strange symmetrical pattern, like two halves of an inkblot.

"There's the brain, in cross section," she said. The image moved, and Susan tracked it expertly, sliding the metal disk across my skin. "Everything looks fine. Now we're going to move down through the body."

I could hardly breathe. The wonder of seeing through myself and the awesome intricacy of the being growing inside me were almost more than I could bear. Several times during my pregnancy I had experienced something miraculous—the Seeing Thing, the hand that had dragged me out of the smoke, the sudden arrival of help when I needed it most. But as I watched the image shift on the ultrasound screen and felt the corresponding movement inside my own body, the miracle of simple reproduction seemed to dwarf them all.

"Larynx is fine," said Susan. She pulled a pen out of her breast pocket and noted something on a clipboard next to the ultrasound machine. "Now we'll go down through the chest."

That machine was truly amazing. A couple of years later, I would have another ultrasound to check on my third child's prenatal development, and it would be nothing like the clarity and specificity of this one. As Susan moved the image through Adam's body, she pointed out all the major organs: lungs, pancreas, stomach, liver, kidneys. She focused in on the heart for some time, and we watched the four chambers pumping out a steady, rapid heartbeat.

"Is it all right?" I asked.

"Looks good," said Susan. "At this stage of development it's sometimes a little hard to tell if all the valves are working correctly. But it looks good."

John was holding my hand very tightly. "Look at that," he breathed. "It may beat for a hundred years." I knew he was as enthralled as I was.

Susan finished making notes on her clipboard. "So," she said. "Do you want a picture of your son?"

"Son?" John and I spoke in unison.

"Oh—I'm sorry." Susan sounded embarrassed. "Didn't you want to know? I thought you already saw—"

"No, no, it's great," I said, my eyes still glued to the ultrasound screen. "A boy."

John squeezed my hand even harder. A flurry of images came into my mind, images of miniature blue jeans, of baseball practice, barbershop haircuts, frogs and snails and puppy-dog tails and every other sentimental cliché that I had ever associated with little boys. I felt tears in my eyes.

"Okay," said Susan warmly. "He's cooperating beautifully. We should be able to get a great snapshot for your photo album." She paused to punch a new set of buttons on the keyboard. Then she slid the transducer around my abdomen, pushing a little to get the right angle.

"And there we go," she said.

I heard John catch his breath. I had stopped breathing altogether. The triangular slice on the ultrasound screen showed a pitch-black background. In the center of it was a clear, bright white profile of a perfectly formed little person. As we watched, our son turned his head slowly, yawned, then put one finger in his mouth and began to suck on it. The other hand reached out, fingers curled into a fist, and pushed against the uterine wall. I could feel the touch of that hand inside me as I watched it on the screen. With my peripheral vision I saw John swipe the cuff of his shirt over his cheek, and I knew he was crying.

I didn't question my own reaction at that instant. I was too riveted by the image on the ultrasound screen. It wasn't until the amniocentesis had been performed and John and I left the clinic that I would begin to wonder about what I thought and felt the first time I saw my baby's face.

The strange thing—the problem, if you want to call it that—was that it *wasn't* the first time. I was positive of that. At the sight of that little face, I was flooded by unmistakable recognition, a sense of déjà vu beyond anything I had ever experienced before. It was like seeing an old friend with a new haircut: he didn't look exactly the way I remembered him, but I definitely remembered him. When I first saw my daughters, I felt the reverent amazement of a discoverer. I was consumed with the desire to get to know them, to find out who they were. When I first saw my son, there on the ultrasound screen, I didn't have this response at all. Instead, I felt the burst of joy that comes when loved ones are reunited, and I thought, "Oh! It's Adam!"

Any way you want to look at it, this was strange. I didn't even know anybody named Adam, nor was it the name we had chosen for the baby. When I was pregnant with Katie, I had briefly considered the name Adam for a boy, because I was looking for soft-sounding consonants to go with Beck, which is one of those clipped Germanic words that sounds absolutely militant when paired with names like Kent or Mitch or Dirk. But I had thought about a thousand names, and Adam was nowhere near the top of the list. John had finally persuaded me that, if we ever did have a boy, we would follow the tradition of the Beck line by naming him after John's Danish-immigrant great-grandfather. The old man's name had been Christen (pronounced "Christian"), and even though I wasn't sure I wanted my son named after a religion, I liked the idea of connecting my children to their Scandinavian ancestry. When I saw Adam on the ultrasound screen, however, there was simply no question of tagging any other name on him. He was Adam, I knew he was Adam, and I'd known him as Adam forever. It was that simple.

During the procedure that followed, I was perplexed and distracted by the intensity of that absolute recognition. The doctor who came in after Susan finished her exam did a much more detailed inspection, measuring skin thickness and comparative bone lengths to add to her data on prenatal diagnosis. She then drew a red X on my abdomen with a Magic Marker and had Susan hold the ultrasound transducer while she pushed a large needle through my skin and into my uterus to withdraw a vial of clear fluid. It was a strange sensation, more like being kicked by a horse than pricked by a pin. John got a little green when he saw the size of the needle, but I didn't focus on it. I was still overwhelmed by encountering my friend Adam after such a long separation, still resonating with the thrum of joy that sang through me when I saw him again, and just beginning to contemplate how irrational, how ridiculous, how impossible this really was.

17

꙳ After the amniocentesis, Susan, the technician, gave us a picture of our baby on a strip of Polaroid paper. I thought Adam was very photogenic. That afternoon we showed the picture to Katie, explaining that it was a portrait of her little brother. I let her put one hand against my side to feel the baby kick while she looked at the picture, trying to make her understand that the image and the strangely active lump in my torso were the same small person. I stuck the picture to the refrigerator door with one of Katie's magnetized letters and taught her to spell "Chris" with some of the others.

John and I were encouraged by the fact that Katie, who was now only a month shy of two years old, seemed fairly interested in playing with the letters. She had already learned to spell "Mom," "Dad," and her own name. True, she had also flushed several of the letters down the toilet, but we felt these were acceptable losses in our quest to raise a literate toddler. Before he left for Asia again, John went out and got a new set to replace the departed portions of the alphabet.

The morning in January when John set out for Singapore again, it was so cold that the engines of his plane wouldn't start. When a replacement aircraft also balked, the pilot told the passengers to go home and wait for the weather to change. John showed up at the apartment about four hours after he'd left, with cracks in the soles of his leather shoes where they had frozen solid and broken as he walked. This is why we now live in Arizona.

I was so happy to see John that I decided to ignore all the work I'd planned for that day. Of course, I would have made the same decision if, for example, there had been a really good episode of *Mister Rogers' Neighborhood* on TV. I had finished writing my term papers, handed them in, and moved on to grading the papers of my students in the Caribbean Society course. After only a few minutes of grading, I came to the realization that as horrible as it is to have to write such papers, it is much more horrible to have to read them. My twenty-four students handed in fifteen pages apiece, meaning that I had to plow through upwards of 350 pages of term paper.

Many of the papers were comparable to decent academic articles, by which I mean that they were factually and grammatically correct, as well as extremely boring. But a considerable number were much worse. They read as if they had been written under intolerable duress, by people in advanced stages of exhaustion and inebriation, who were trying desperately to appear to know more than they did. The reason was that this was exactly how they *were* written. I was pretty sure of this because a couple of years earlier, when I was an undergraduate, that's exactly how I and all my friends had written our term papers. My last paper as a graduating senior was written on my fourth consecutive night without sleep. I had to write very short sentences because my brain was retaining phrases of only five words or less. I would forget, right in the middle of typing a phrase, what the paper was about, and what the sentence was supposed to say. May God have mercy on the soul of the poor teaching fellow who had to read that one.

A few days after John finally did take off for Singapore, leaving me with now-familiar feelings of isolation and vulnerability, I forced myself through the last of the term papers. Most of the really awful ones focused on reggae, a style of music that originated in Jamaica and had many avid fans among the students in the Caribbean Society course. Reggae is heavily associated with marijuana use, which may account for the bizarre syntax and faint weedy aroma that lingered on many of the pages. As I read them, my family's battle cry of "What an idiot!" rang through my consciousness many, many times. I tried to rein Fang back and grade the papers fairly, writing the kind of supportive criticism I would have wanted to receive myself. Then I handed the papers back, turned in my grades, and thought I was finished.

Hah.

I don't know if Harvard students argue their grades any more vociferously than students at any other university. It does seem likely, however, that the place attracts a disproportionate share of the kinds of folks who would rather take a teaching fellow hostage than accept a low mark. Almost as soon as I'd handed the papers back, I was besieged by students wanting to come speak to me about their grades. This meant that instead of whiling away the days of John's absence eating leftover Christmas bonbons and watching my stomach grow, I had to show up at my office every day and wrangle with people who were not pleased with me, oh no, not at all.

After a couple of days, it began to get to me. Once again, I felt as though I had nearly emptied my small stores of energy and something drastic was going to happen if I didn't get more rest. This infuriated me. I wasn't accustomed to cutting corners professionally just because I felt awful. One of my favorite Harvard stories (very apropos at grading time) concerned a student who handed in a paper late, explaining to his professor that he hadn't been able to finish it on time because he wasn't feeling well. The professor responded, "My boy, you will find that most of the great deeds in human history were accomplished by people who weren't feeling well." Needless to say, the student got a very low grade. The professor went on to become the president of Harvard.

I reminded myself of this story on the seventh day of John's January trip, as I dragged myself to my office to hear more grievances from my students. The first person to visit my office that morning threatened to kill herself unless I changed her B+ to an A. The next told me that she had decided to use the Caribbean Society class not to learn about Caribbean society but to come to terms with her complete lack of interest in the subject. She had written a paper about why she hadn't read any of the text material or attended the lectures, and she felt she deserved an A for introspection. A third student had produced a lively, well-written discussion of Caribbean history, which would have been an A paper if any of the events he mentioned—wars, elections, droughts, plagues— had ever really happened. When I explained that historical treatises work best when they are related to actual facts, the student burst out, "I didn't come to Harvard to regurgitate facts! I came here to learn to think *creatively!*" I had to admire the boldness of his position, but even in my state of diminishing mental acuity, it seemed to me there were some flaws in the logic.

Things went on this way until it was time to pick Katie up and go back to the apartment. Walking over to the day-care center, I could tell something was seriously wrong. I had long since accepted that I would never feel great while I was pregnant, but this was different. I was disoriented and extremely weak. I felt as though there were a dreadful struggle taking place inside me. Much later, during my third pregnancy, this feeling would come over me again. At that point, under close medical supervision, I would learn that my hyperactive immune system was reacting to the fetus in my womb as though it were a foreign object, like a transplanted organ that didn't match my genetic code. I was having a severe toxic reaction. At the time, I didn't know this. All I knew was that I wasn't feeling well, and, as we all know, most of the great deeds in human history were accomplished by people who weren't feeling well.

Right now, my great deeds were pretty much limited to putting on Katie's snowsuit, hat, mittens, and boots, and helping her into her backpack. The normal procedure at that point was to set the pack down on a table or desk, with Katie in it, and slide my arms through the straps. I did get that far, but when I stood up and took Katie's weight on my shoulders, I nearly collapsed. I backed up and set the pack down again. Then I slid Katie out of it and told her we would walk home together that day.

It took us about an hour to cover the mile to the apartment. It was snowing heavily, and the fresh powder rested on a layer of slick ice that coated the uneven cobblestones. We both fell down a lot. Every time I hit the snow, I had more serious doubts about getting up. But eventually I would grit my teeth, remind myself of the Harvard president and his sluggish student, and get back on my feet.

Looking back, I am amazed at how flat-out stupid I was not to acknowledge, or even recognize, my body's desperate attempts to communicate to me that something was seriously wrong. The only self-defense I have is that our entire society celebrates people who push themselves to extremes, who force themselves onward through pain, fatigue, and injury to achieve all kinds of improbable objectives. The message of a million cultural icons, from sports heroes to movie characters, is that if you could just try a little harder, bear a little more agony, ignore a little more of your desire to quit, you would be fabulously rich and successful and get away from the bad guys every time.

As we wended our slippery way home, I thought about the week Katie was born. I was just finishing a project I'd been doing for a well-known psychology professor, making a series of drawings for him to use in an experiment on human perception. My labor started two days before the drawings were due. As soon as I realized that the birth was imminent, I began to work frenziedly, determined not to let myself be sidetracked. I wasn't going to be a wimpy antifeminist who stops her career dead in its tracks at the birth of her first child. No, I was going to be a much stauncher woman, one of the sort who politely excuse themselves for a minute or two, go behind a bush to deliver, and come back a few minutes later with babies strapped to their backs to pick up work where they left off. I kept working on those drawings until my contractions were so intense and frequent that I couldn't hold a pencil steady.

The labor lasted halfway through the day on which the drawings were due. After Katie was born, I slept for six hours, asked to be released from the hospital, took the baby home, and handed her over to my mother, who had just flown in from Utah. Then I sat up all night finishing the drawings. I only held Katie long enough to feed her. Each time I did it, I had to muster all my willpower to force myself to hand her back to my mother. Every cell in my body resisted letting go of that tiny, warm, miraculous little body. When morning broke, I put on a huge down coat of John's (to hide the distressing facts that my abdomen hadn't snapped immediately back to normal and that each of my breasts had suddenly grown larger than my head), and doggedly trudged a mile to the psychology professor's office.

"These are late," he said when I handed him the pictures.

"I know," I said. "I apologize. I went into labor."

He glanced at me. "You don't look like you're in labor."

"I'm not. I had a baby."

"Oh," he grunted and went back to peering at the pictures. He pointed out a few flaws and asked for some changes. I noted them. We set another date when the corrected final product would be due, and I trudged home again. Nothing further was said about the fact that I'd just given birth.

The feeling I had as I walked away from that psychology professor's office was the same feeling that seized me almost two years later, as Katie and I slowly covered the same route from William James Hall to our apartment—an immense, aching emptiness. Right after having Katie, I had assumed that it was merely the huge, aching emptiness of my uterus, which had been through a lot over the previous few days and was used to having more company. When I was expecting Adam, this clearly was not the problem. It seems utterly obvious to me now that the terrible yearning I felt was the call of every part of myself except my intellect—body, heart, and soul—trying desperately to get me to listen to them.

Of course I didn't. I was doing my best to follow the example of the action hero who charges onward despite the bullets lodged in every limb, the dancer who leaps through six hours of rehearsal on nothing but breath mints and willpower, the athlete who wins the championship by ignoring injuries that will ultimately cripple him for life.

It absolutely amazes me that I was so proud of my own inner deafness. It's like being proud to say that you've gone to the Grand Canyon and refused to look at the scenery, focusing instead on something like a bottle cap or a blown-out truck tire. I am no longer proud that during my daughter's first day of life I forfeited holding her in order to finish some trivial project for some trivial experiment. I'm not proud that I spent years dulling any impulse that did not motivate me to work. And I am not proud that I forced myself to keep walking, refusing to call for any help, on that afternoon when Katie and I inched our way home from the day-care center.

When we got there it was almost five o'clock, already dark. There were two messages on the answering machine, one from John and one from Sibyl. Ever since the day she had shown up at my apartment, Sibyl had quietly persisted in checking to make sure I was all right—especially when John was away. She had brought me food more times than I could count, offered me a lift in her car whenever she knew I needed it, and often brought Mie over on weekends to brighten my day and make Katie's. When I returned her phone call that night, I could have told her that for some reason I was too weak to help Katie off with her snowsuit. Knowing Sibyl, she would not have rested until I was under a doctor's care and feeling considerably better.

Of course, that is exactly why I forced myself not to mention how rotten I felt. I was determined not to be a burden yet again. When I spoke to Sibyl, I was careful to inject some cheeriness into my voice. I told her everything was fine. Then I hung up the phone and burst into tears. That inner voice was screaming now, begging me to get some kind of assistance. I clamped my jaw and reminded myself that I was strong, I was invincible, I was woman. Years later, while reading Chinese philosophy, I would stumble across the Taoist saying that "when two great forces collide, the victory will go to the one that knows how to yield." The idea is that a fluid substance, like water, may seem to give in to a rigid substance, like stone—but in the end, it is the water that shapes the stone, and not the other way around. That evening in Cambridge, I was deliberately trying to turn myself to stone.

I talked Katie through the removal of her winter wear and managed to change her diaper. We watched a videotaped version of *Sesame Street* while Katie ate a peanut butter sandwich and drained her bottle. Then we both fell asleep on the futon without even undressing.

I slipped immediately into a series of terrible dreams. I dreamt about my next-door neighbor, the woman who had seized my wrist during the fire and begged me to get her out of the building. I dreamt that Katie was drowning in the sea and that I, for some reason, was refusing to go to the rescue. I dreamt that John came home, but as I reached to embrace him, his body grew transparent and began to vanish from within my arms.

I woke up, covered with sweat, at about 2:00 A.M. I was incredibly tired. My heart was hammering, and I felt curiously breathless. I lay there for a few minutes, watching the lights of cars and storefronts reflected on the apartment ceiling from the icy streets ten stories down. There was an uncomfortable buzzing in my ears. I was extremely cold. I put out my hand to make sure Katie was covered by the quilt and felt a wet spot between us on the bed. I sighed. I hadn't changed her diaper again before she fell asleep. I patted her bottom to gauge the wetness of the diaper and was confused to find it quite dry. I felt the wet spot on the bed again and discovered that it was spreading around *me*. Oh, this was just great. Not only did I feel like dog chow, not only had I become Our Lady of Perpetual Nausea, but now I had lost bladder control. I could hardly wait to find out what new indignities awaited me as my pregnancy continued.

I was tired, unbelievably tired, much too tired to change the sheets, let alone do the laundry. I decided that I would just change my clothes, cover the wet spot with a towel, and clean up in the morning.

The buzzing in my ears got dramatically louder as I headed toward the bathroom, panting rapidly. I had the kind of head rush you get when you stand up too fast after a few glasses of wine, except that this one went on and on and on. I also felt even more disoriented than I had earlier that afternoon. That was why, when I got to the bathroom and started taking off my clothes, I didn't even register that anything unusual was happening. I kept my enormous pregnancy sweater on as I peeled off my blue jeans and the long underwear that helped me handle the New England cold. I don't remember noticing anything unusual about them. It was only when I turned to wash my hands, and saw that the water running down the drain looked strangely rusty, that I finally realized that my hands—along with my jeans, my long johns, my legs, and the bed in the other room—were covered with bright red blood.

18

When Adam was about a year old and could sit up well on his own, I used to let him take baths with Katie. They had many grand times, splashing water into each other's faces and coating the tile with soap slime. One day, while I was bathing the children, I smelled smoke and realized that a pot of spaghetti sauce I had left on the stove was boiling over. It had, in fact, started a small fire. I rushed to the kitchen and began smothering the flames. John, who had been working in his office, was only seconds behind me. As we doused the flames, we began to snap at each other about whose responsibility it was to cook dinner that night.

Right in the middle of this rather testy exchange, both of us suddenly shut up. John says that at that moment a vivid image flashed into his mind; an image of Adam facedown in the bathwater. At the same instant, I heard a voice in my head—a very insistent one—say, *"Check the tub!"*

I turned and ran the short distance to the bathroom. As I neared the door, I heard Katie's small, bemused voice saying, "Adam, wake up! Adam, why won't you wake up? Adam?"

Adam was floating facedown, just as John had "seen" him. His little body was the color of lilacs. I began to scream uncontrollably as I lifted him out of the five inches of water—more than enough, as I now know, to kill a child—and John ran to the phone to dial 911. He was so panicked that instead he kept dialing 411, which of course is directory assistance. The operator kept coming on and saying, "What city?" John kept shouting into the phone, "There's a drowned child here! My son is drowning!" Eventually, he managed to dial the right number, and a team of paramedics immediately set out for our house.

They would not have arrived in time. Adam wasn't breathing at all when I picked him up. His body was as floppy and lifeless as so much rubber. But even as I continued to scream, the silent voice that had alerted me to the danger in the first place began to give me quick, clear instructions. My body followed them with eerie calm, as though it were under the control of someone far more self-assured. I put Adam down on his back, blew air into his nose and mouth, then turned his head to one side and pressed gently on his sternum. After five or six repetitions of this procedure, a gush of water bubbled out of Adam's lungs, and he drew a shallow breath. I screamed one more time, *"He's breathing!"* and kept up the mouth-to-mouth resuscitation until Adam opened his eyes, blinked, and gave me a tremulous smile. I had done exactly what I was taught to do in an infant CPR course—several weeks later. At the time Adam nearly drowned, I wasn't trained in CPR. The Bunraku puppeteers apparently were.

The fact that I was able to save Adam's life assuaged some of my guilt at having been so stupid as to leave him in the bathtub with only a three-year-old's supervision. I eventually managed to forgive myself, although I had a hard time letting my children go near water for a long time. (Until they learned to take showers, which is not easy for a toddler, they were notable for their grubbiness.) The feeling that lasted longest after the drowning incident was not guilt but the stabbing realization of how precious Adam was to me, how much my life is lightened by his presence, and how lost I would be without the angels he brings with him, as my friend says, the way a dog brings fleas. For the awful minute or two that I thought my son was dead, I wasn't feeling sorry for him. I was feeling sorry for me.

I had exactly the same reaction the January before Adam was born, in another bathroom, when I saw the blood on my hands and legs and realized that my pregnancy might end a lot sooner than I'd expected. I've read articles on obstetrical technologies that mention how much more difficult it is for a woman to lose a baby after seeing it on an ultrasound screen, and it's true that the snapshot of Adam on our refrigerator made him seem more real to me. But I wasn't simply attached to a generic baby, which is pretty much what Adam looked like in the picture. I had the same feeling about my son, already, that I had about anyone else I deeply loved. I knew him. I *felt* him, the way you feel any loved one's presence when you are together, even when no words are spoken. I don't know if it

was because of the strange experiences that began when Adam was conceived, or the dreams I'd been having, or some sort of metaphysical connection, but I had an almost tangible sense of my son's personality, his
unique and indestructible identity. The idea of losing him was simply
unthinkable.

I sat down on the closed toilet, telling myself not to worry. If I'd
known why I was bleeding, I would have told myself to go right ahead
and worry—a *lot*. The blood was coming from what is known as a placental abruption, a condition in which the placenta, which conducts nu-
trients from a mother's bloodstream to her unborn baby, tears away from
the wall of the uterus. This rarely happens unless a pregnant woman un-
dergoes some dramatic physical trauma, like a car accident in which various auto parts are rammed directly into her torso. After Adam was born,
several people—including some doctors—assumed that the problem
must have been caused by his Down syndrome. However, exactly the
same thing would happen two years later, during my third pregnancy,
when the baby was as normal as pie. My gut feeling (if you'll pardon the
pun) is that I had these placental abruptions because of the autoimmune
condition that made me so violently nauseated. I guess I'll never know
for certain.

Anyway, because the placenta is so rich in blood vessels, a placental
abruption is a very serious condition indeed. The fetus dies in most cases,
and the mother can also bleed to death in a matter of minutes, depend-
ing on how much of the placenta has separated from the uterine wall.
Medical science can't do much about it, beyond giving transfusions to
save the mother's life. Of course, I didn't know any of this as I groggily
washed the blood off my hands in the middle of that New England night,
feeling like Lady Macbeth with a bad hangover. I was a little shaky about
the baby, but the idea that *I* might die of pregnancy-related causes never
even occurred to me.

I'd like to say that at this point I calmly phoned for medical assistance, then tidied up my bloodstained apartment while waiting for the
ambulance to arrive. But the truth is that I panicked like a gut-shot deer.
My heart began to race, and my hands started shaking violently with

what felt like cold but may have been shock. I had just enough pragma-
tism left to install a maxi pad and wipe some of the blood off my legs and
hands. When I stood up, I caught a glimpse of my face in the bathroom
mirror. I looked as though I'd been made up for Halloween. My skin was
fish-belly white except for my freckles, which never completely go away
even in winter, and my lips, which were a bluish shade of mauve. As I
started toward the bedroom my ears began to ring, a sound that quickly
escalated into an unpleasant rasping hum.

Back in my bedroom, Katie was sleeping peacefully on the futon, her
curly blond hair and fringe of black eyelashes making her look like a
Baroque cherub. She didn't wake up when I turned on the bedside lamp
and started shuffling through the stacks of books I kept by the bed. I
found my favorite, a fairly dense medical textbook. My hands were trembling so hard that I barely managed to look up "bleeding" in the index.
Some part of my brain kept telling me that this had to be normal, that
somewhere in my reference books I'd find a calming explanation for co-
pious blood loss in the fifth month of pregnancy. It wasn't there. There
were a few references to bleeding, but none of them sounded like what
was happening to me, and all of them were bad. I closed the book and
tried to put it back on the night table, but my grip was weak and my fingers were numb and I dropped it on the floor. Instead of picking it up, I
pulled my hands back in to my stomach, trying desperately to hold the
baby inside me, to protect him. I absolutely refused to let him die. Not
now. Not after everything we'd been through together.

The humming in my ears was getting louder. I've read accounts of
near-death experiences in which people report hearing a buzzing sound
just before they were declared dead, and although I don't think I was all
that close to expiring, sometimes I wonder if they are talking about the
same rasping hum I heard that night. My head was beginning to ache. I
wanted desperately to just lie down and fall asleep, to escape whatever
was happening to my body. Still, somewhere in my jumbled brain a tiny
molecule of reason shrilled at me to call the obstetrician. I found the
phone, dialed, and got the answering service for UHS. They said they
would page the doctor on call.

I managed to get the phone back onto its cradle and curled up on the bed again, still wearing my heavy sweater, to wait for the doctor's call. I was freezing. My hands and feet were completely numb, and my teeth wouldn't stop chattering. Katie had kicked off the small flannel blanket I'd spread over her. I reached over to replace it, but she rolled away, still sleeping soundly. I touched her head and was surprised to find that she was warm, her hair slightly damp with sweat. I couldn't even remember what warm felt like. The cold seemed to have seeped right into my marrow. I pulled the baby blanket over myself and tried to relax.

By the time the phone rang, the humming in my ears had crescendoed into a roar. It almost drowned out the sound of the doctor's voice on the other end of the line.

"H'llo," I said through my chattering teeth.

The doctor introduced himself. The obstetricians who dealt with Harvard worked in rotations. This was someone I'd never met.

"So," said the doctor, "what seems to be the problem?"

"Well, I seem to be pregnant," I said, trying to sound jocular, "and I seem to be bleeding."

He didn't laugh. "How far along are you?" he said.

"About twenty weeks. Five months."

"Okay," said the doctor. "How much blood is there?"

I looked at the stain on the bedsheets and felt a trickle of fluid on my leg. "Not a whole bunch," I said. "Nothing you could fill a bucket with, or anything like that. But it got all over my clothes."

"What color is it?" the doctor asked. "Is it a brownish color, or bright red?"

"Um, bright," I said, my teeth clicking like castanets. "Very bright red."

I could hear him take a deep breath and let it out again.

"Okay, Mrs. Beck," he said. "You need to get to the emergency room as soon as possible."

I closed my eyes. The thought of getting anywhere, especially anywhere outside the bedroom, brought on a wave of exhaustion. I almost fell asleep right then and there.

"Mrs. Beck?"

I jumped a little, startled by his voice. "Uh-huh," I said.

"Have your husband drive you to the emergency room, okay? Right now. The sooner the better."

I frowned, rubbing my free hand over my eyes. I could have explained to the doctor that my husband wasn't around, that I didn't have a car, that I couldn't leave Katie alone, and that taking her with me in a taxi in the middle of this freezing night was utterly beyond my capability. Anyway, I could barely hear the doctor over that awful noise in my ears.

"Mrs. Beck? Are you there?"

I was irritated by the question. I didn't want to answer any more questions. I felt as though I were sinking into a deep, black pool. A cold one.

"I'm coming, I'm coming," I said irritably.

"All right," said the doctor. "Hurry."

I hung up and put my hands over my ears to block the buzzing sound. It didn't work. I could feel more blood on my leg, but I didn't have the energy to get up and install a new pad. I understood at some level that the doctor would not have told me to go to the emergency room unless something was really wrong, but I simply couldn't imagine getting to the hospital. I could sense my connection to the physical world slipping away, drop by drop by drop.

As it did, however, I began to notice them.

The more my normal perceptions waned, the more clearly I understood that there were other presences in the room besides me and Katie. It was like watching rocks and stumps emerge from the sea as the tide pulls back, exposing them to the daylight. Of course, I had been aware of the Bunraku puppeteers for months—but I had never quite let go of my disbelief in them. It was always "as if": I felt *as if* there were people watching me, *as if* small miracles were happening, *as if* some force I could not see were conveying messages between me and the people I loved. On the night I started bleeding, the as if's melted away. I could not physically see or hear the beings in that room, but their presence was as real and ordinary to me as the presence of oxygen. There must have been eight or ten of them, standing in the bedroom, looking on with great concern as I grew weaker and the roaring in my ears got louder. Somehow, their presence allowed me to realize the extent of my illness, and my fear. I felt a sob force its way up my throat.

"You guys," I whispered to the beings in the room. "Help this baby."

It was the first time I had spoken to them directly. In doing so, I felt myself cross a fine but very distinct line, the line between speculating about the existence of a metaphysical plane of some sort and climbing aboard for the ride. I knew I had let go of my sanity. It was terrifying. I only did it because my fear of what was happening to my body had become greater than my fear of holding on to irrational beliefs.

As soon as I asked them to help the baby, I felt a flood of warmth rush through my torso. It was extremely soothing, as intense as it was brief. The bleeding stopped instantly. I knew it. I knew it the same way that I knew the beings were there. Then the warmth was gone, leaving me aching with cold, dizzy with blood loss, and as scared as ever. I ran my tongue over my lips, which might as well have been filled with Novocain.

"Please," I said, feeling strange and awkward, like Oliver Twist asking for more porridge, "please help me, too."

For some reason, saying this was one of the hardest things I have ever done. I felt a crushing combination of swallowed pride and unworthiness, along with that sense that I was walking deliberately into irrational territory.

The response was immediate. It came in a form I had already experienced, that night in Sibyl and Charles's house after the fire. First, a hand—or in this case a set of hands—seemed to reach out of the air and catch me, like a father catching a falling child. One hand went around my back to support me, while another rested flat on my chest, across my collarbone. That incredibly soothing warmth emanated from the hands into my body.

You'd think that at this point I would have been transported in some kind of holy rapture, like Bernadette communing with the Virgin Mary. Not me. I'm afraid I'm just not saint material. As the warmth from those two strong hands flowed into me that night, bringing me a few inches out of my numbed, bloodless daze, I did not just praise the Lord and relax. Instead, I found myself bothered by something about those hands. The problem was that they were *male*. Like all little children in Utah, I had been thoroughly saturated throughout my tender years with images of God as a bearded Caucasian gentleman with X-ray vision and a touchy disposition. I didn't like that image as a child, I rejected it as an adolescent, and I was perversely peeved to have it reinforced, in any way, that night in Cambridge.

"What do you know about being pregnant?" I grumbled to the owner of those wonderfully warm hands.

I didn't have to explain what I meant. I knew I had been heard. I didn't believe a male, of whatever plasmic density, could understand what I was going through at that moment. I wanted someone who had been through it, someone who had felt torn to shreds by the process of creating life, by having to decide between her own welfare and the welfare of the child inside her, between the care of the living child and the child yet to be born. The horror of that night was not so much my fear of death as my realization that I didn't have enough resources to let us all— me, Katie, and the little boy whose picture was taped to the refrigerator door—survive. I was facing an intolerable choice. I felt wounded by that struggle in a way that went beyond physical pain, and I did not merely want to be fixed. I wanted—I needed—to be *understood*.

As soon as this thought came into my mind, the hands that had been touching me pulled back, leaving me freezing and falling into the darkness. Before I even had time to register another wave of fear, a second pair of hands replaced the first. I could feel them stroking my forehead and pressing softly against my abdomen. They touched me the way an experienced groom touches a panicked horse, gently but with great authority. These hands were smaller than the first set, narrow and quick as well as very strong. They were definitely a woman's hands. And in my head, without really hearing anything, I had the impression that this female being was saying to me, "Well, it took you long enough to ask!"

The twilight zone I reached that night, the region between my world and the world of those invisible helpers, was a place where certainty and uncertainty seemed to be reversed. I was unsure of everything that was happening to me physically, but I took for granted a great many things that I would have disbelieved at any normal moment. Not only did I know that those incorporeal beings were there, but it was utterly clear to me that the only reason they hadn't been helping me all along, taking out the garbage and delinting the couch and so on, was that I hadn't wanted them to. They wouldn't—they couldn't—do anything for me until I asked. And I had to *mean it.* When I finally did ask, I opened the cosmic door an inch or so, but I opened it to the only image of God I had ever encountered: God as a man. Once I asked for a woman, *shazzam,* they could send a woman. I felt very strongly that the one thing these beings would never do, under any circumstances, was override my will.

I don't know what they were. The word *angel* never occurred to me at the time. Neither did *ghost, spirit,* or any of the other terms ordinarily used to describe such intangible visitors. Even now, thinking back on it, I don't know what I would call them. They could have been emissaries from the Spiral Nebula for all I know. The only word that comes to mind when I remember that night is *friend.* They were my friends, and they loved me, and that was all that mattered at the time.

Isn't it possible, you may well be thinking, that I imagined these beings? After all, I was dehydrated, had lost a good deal of blood, and was definitely thinking-impaired. My answer to this question is a resounding yes. It makes good sense to me that the human brain would cook up a few reassuring fantasies in conditions of extreme duress. For years after Adam was born, I tried almost frantically to figure out *exactly* what was happening on occasions like this one. For now, suffice it to say that any way you want to explain "paranormal" experiences like this, from blaming them on delusion to believing they are being broadcast live from the Hale-Bopp comet, is fine with me. The only thing I can tell you is what I experienced.

Whatever they were, wherever they came from, whomever they belonged to, the hands kept touching me, sending that sublimely comforting warmth gradually through my skin and into my muscle and bone. They calmed my intense, animal fear, replacing it with the security of a baby being rocked to sleep. I knew that my little boy and I were both out of danger. The same spent relief came over me that I would feel more than a year later when Adam coughed and gurgled and came to life again after his misadventure in the bathtub.

Slowly, slowly, as those small, strong hands radiated healing into my body, I began to trust these beings whose presence had shadowed my life for the past months. At a certain point, without really articulating it, I silently agreed to accept any and all help they were willing to give me. The man's hands immediately joined the woman's. Then another pair joined the two of them, and then another, and another, until there seemed to be a whole gang of them around me, putting that gentle pressure against my body. I did not "fall" into sleep that night. I rose into it, out of the black, cold pool, as though I were being lifted by a thousand wings.

19

I woke up to the ringing of the telephone. It was nearly noon.

The voice on the other end belonged to the obstetrician I had spoken to earlier, in the wee hours of the morning. He was very worried. He had gone off shift a few minutes after speaking with me, and when he came back to work, he was shocked to find that I hadn't ever arrived at the emergency room.

I told the doctor I was fine and thanked him for his trouble. This didn't satisfy him. He wouldn't hang up until I promised to at least go over to the clinic to have a doctor check me out. I swore on a stack of Bibles that I would. I lied.

There were two reasons I didn't go over to University Health Services that morning. The first was that I associated the place, above all, with having blood taken. It seemed to me that the nurses there drew liters of my blood every time I went in, even if I was only dropping off some paperwork. That morning, my large veins were flat and limp, and I was churlishly possessive about every drop of blood I had left. But equally important, I stayed away from UHS because I was utterly, illogically certain that the bleeding had stopped, that the baby and I were both fine. I could feel Adam kicking away, but the reason for my perverse certainty came from something even deeper inside me. I could have told the doctor, "Lo, verily, I have been healed," but I couldn't even articulate this to myself without fearing for my sanity.

There was a kind of braced sensation in my body, as though my tissues were being held together by stronger material than had been available to them for several months. Even so, I crept around the apartment rather gingerly for a while, one hand plastered to my abdomen to feel the baby's reassuring movements. Katie had apparently been awake for some time, sucking absentmindedly on her bottle and playing with a set of educational blocks John and I had bought her for Christmas. I changed her diaper, got her some crackers and fruit to go with the bottle, and switched on *Sesame Street*, her true primary caretaker. Then I turned my attention to feeding myself.

For the first time since I got pregnant, I actually wanted to eat. In fact, I had an immense and highly specific craving for two things: hot tea and sirloin steak. In the weeks since Food Shak burned down, John and I had discovered the highly expensive wonders of grocery-store delivery. I called a nearby store and ordered several pounds of sirloin. I already had a couple of stray tea bags in a box at the back of a kitchen cupboard. I brewed and guzzled about a quart of it, enjoying it immensely.

When the intercom buzzed, I welcomed the grocery delivery boy with the enthusiasm of a cave woman seizing fresh kill from a passing Neanderthal. He seemed surprised that I was alone—I think he had assumed I was in the middle of some gala barbecue for a houseful of farmhands. I tipped him liberally, then set to work cooking and scarfing down more red meat than I had eaten in the previous year. Ordinarily, I avoid caffeine and meat, not because I'm trying to be virtuous but because I don't like them. But my blood supply was intent on rebuilding itself, and to that end I had suddenly become devoutly carnivorous. Wonder of wonders, the steak and tea actually seemed to lighten my nausea. They instantly became my favorite foods. For the last half of that pregnancy I would subsist almost entirely on Earl Grey and sirloin, with an occasional sixteen-ounce bar of Belgian chocolate thrown in for variety. (Watch for my new health and fitness best-seller, *Eight Weeks to Cardiac Arrest*.)

It wasn't until I had finished my last hunk of steak, dressed Katie, and taken a shower that I set out to face the fact that there were invisible people in my apartment.

I had pushed the memory of the previous night into the same half-conscious area of my mind where I stored the rescue from the smoke-filled staircase and the reassuring touch I had felt in Sibyl's apartment. So far I hadn't allowed either event into full awareness, because I didn't know what to do with them. I was afraid of the ramifications. Incorporeal hands did not fit into life as I knew it. They weren't something I could simply dismiss as pleasantly unusual, like bumping into an old friend in an unfamiliar place. The whole thing was a huge, bright, mystifying, terrifying conundrum.

The first thing I did was to take a notebook and a pen and slowly, methodically write down every thought, sight, sound, and sensation I had experienced the previous night. Then I reread the account several times, as if it were a psychotic letter I'd received from a previously sane acquaintance ("Yes, Officer, she was always quiet and kept mostly to herself, although lately she'd begun ordering all this meat . . ."). It would almost have been easier for me if I'd been able to believe I was hallucinating, but although I knew I *could* have been delusional, I couldn't honestly say that I *believed* I was. On the one hand, to dismiss the visitors as figments of my imagination would have been a lie. On the other hand, to say that they were real would rock my worldview to its foundation. I reread my account of my own experiences over and over, unable to live with either interpretation.

I decided to take it in stages. I stopped focusing on figuring out what these visitors were and turned my attention to the epiphany they had brought with them, the one in which I realized that they would never override my power to make my own decisions. Until that moment, I had felt caught up in a great tidal wave of forces stronger than myself: the primeval urge to procreate, the uncontrollable changes in my own body, the need for John to build his career even if it meant long absences, and above all, the towering nightmare of requirements necessary to succeed at Harvard. The morning after the bleeding incident it suddenly seemed obvious—as it still does—that every one of these things had much less power over me than my own ability to choose. My responses to my pregnancy, to my own bad health, to John's career choices, to the requirements of school and work, were entirely under my own command. This left me nearly breathless with responsibility but also awed and exhilarated by freedom. I had to get up and pace around the apartment, trying to let it sink in.

The realization that I was the captain of my own fate had some frightening implications. For instance, was I now responsible for acknowledging my new belief system to people at Harvard? I tried to think of ways I could defend myself from the criticism I would draw if I did. Every step forward in human knowledge, I told myself, looks and sounds insane to everyone but the people who discover it. But I knew how well that one would go over in the Ivy League. After all, thinking there are invisible people in your bedroom does not sound like a step forward in human knowledge. If anything, it's a step *backward*, to the time when everyone assumed illness was caused by demonic possession and bad luck always denoted divine disfavor.

I had been raised around people who believed such things, devout Mormons who would credit God and angels with just about everything that ever happened to them. For example, when I was little my family knew a woman who was so enormously fat that one day she got stuck going through her kitchen door. The woman's entire family prayed for her release from the doorframe, until finally, with a great heave, she popped loose and headed on into the kitchen, presumably to get something to eat. Another acquaintance had actually arranged for a neighbor, who was not Mormon, to care for her pet ducks after Jesus came again, since she (the Mormon) was going to be caught up to heaven, while her neighbor would be left behind with all the other sinners.

I had spent most of my life trying to disassociate myself from such people. It had not been easy. My parents were Mormon, though by no means typical; they believed in a strange blend of religion and intellectualism that had made me a childhood pariah among both my Mormon and my non-Mormon peers. All the neighbors and the kids at school believed in a sort of Republican, apple-pie-eating God, whose primary concern was that we all live exactly like the von Trapp family in *The Sound of Music*. My parents, by contrast, believed in a God who backed the Democrats in every election and whose pet peeves were brainless evangelism and kitschy art of any genre. In Utah, children take each other's views of Divinity very seriously. I got beaten up regularly in elementary school because of my fidelity to my parents' God. By sixth grade, I—or rather, Fang—had become a "problem child" who made Sunday school teachers cry with her scalding sarcasm.

By the time I left for Harvard, I was an atheist. I had come to agree with Albert Camus that the only significant decision left in a godless universe was whether or not to commit suicide. The decision was pretty close to a toss-up for me. It had weighed so heavily on my mind that I took the next year off from Harvard and read a lot of Western philosophy, from the pre-Socratics to the postmodernists. Then I read the basic texts of several world religions and finished off with a layperson's tour of theoretical physics. I was looking, in case you haven't guessed, for the Meaning of Life. I couldn't find it.

I did come out of that year with a new life philosophy, a kind of skeptical relativism that allowed me to operate in the diametrically opposing environments of my Harvard education and my Mormon heritage. The bedrock of this worldview was the fact that no version of reality is ultimately testable. In other words, while there was no way for my family's bulky acquaintance to prove that Jesus shoved her through the kitchen door, there was also no way for me to prove that he didn't. I respected my family and friends' religious beliefs, in a detached, social-sciency sort of way, while secretly believing that faith in God was not only the opiate of the masses but the refuge of people too craven to accept the fact of their own mortality. In short, I belonged to the same religion as everyone else I knew at Harvard.

I began to wonder if my experiences during the night meant that the deeply religious people who had peopled my childhood were actually, empirically *right*. The thought made me shudder. Fang rose up from the left side of my brain, snarling and disdainful. "Fantasy!" she said. "Wishful thinking! Hallucinatory brain spasms!"

This sounded reasonable to me. "That's right," I thought, breathing a little easier—but just then Adam landed a solid kick to my kidneys, and I was struck all over again by amazement at what was happening to me.

Over the course of two or three days, I gradually revised my own conception of reality. I did not come to any firm conclusions. Instead, I decided on a major change in the way I would position my investigation. Until that point, I had followed the good old Baconian logic of refusing to believe anything until it was proven true. Now I decided that I was willing to believe anything, absolutely anything I heard, saw, or felt, until it was proven *false*. If this doesn't sound like a major life transition to you, it's because you've never done it. With this single decision, I expanded my reality from a string of solid facts, as narrow, strong, and cold as a razor's edge, to a wild chaos of possibility.

When John returned from Singapore at the end of that week, he looked different—not because he had changed but because I had. It was strange to see my husband with the new vision I had developed, strange to see that he looked exactly the same, and that I was as crazy about him as ever. He became very worried when I told him about the bleeding incident. He would have dragged me over to the health clinic then and there, if it had been up to him. I told him I was fine. I almost said that I *knew* I was healed, because, see, these invisible people had made a house call to our apartment and fixed me right up, just when things had been looking a little bleak. The urge to tell him everything and the fear that he'd think I was crazy battled inside me with considerable force, but in the end my fear of ridicule won out.

This might seem strange in light of the fact that John, like every teenage boy who grew up in our hometown, had gone out to serve a Mormon mission when he was nineteen. That was how he'd fallen in love with Asia and become fluent in Japanese. But John's religious views were, if anything, less faith-directed than mine. Whereas I viewed my religion as a sort of ethnic heritage, like being born Jewish, John saw Mormonism primarily as a useful social institution, good for keeping children off the streets and adults out of prison. He was not into mysticism, or even the kind of existential crisis I had been through as a young adult. Such things would have been considered very inappropriate in his family context. He had followed his parents' religious standards primarily because anything else would have looked disgraceful to the neighbors.

The difference in our basic worldviews was the one subject we had never been able to talk about with any degree of comfort. You'd think it would be essential for a married couple to discuss such things, but we had always wordlessly agreed that issues of faith would be a demilitarized zone between us, a place where all comment and interaction were forbidden. The life of the spirit was more personal, more vulnerable, more embarrassing a topic than sex or politics or emotion. It was territory we had never been in together. We would both go a long way into that territory—separate, isolated, and bewildered—before the journey would finally become too difficult and frightening, too comforting and beautiful, to bear alone.

20

John was one tired hombre. He'd been living on opposite sides of the globe for almost five months, trying to get so much done that it would seem he was actually living full-time in both places. In pictures of him that were taken that year, he looks older than he does today. His circadian rhythm, the rise and fall of temperature and other functions that was supposed to tell his body when to eat, sleep, work, and move, was thoroughly and miserably out of sync.

Since his latest return home, John kept reaching over to touch me, as if to reassure himself that I wasn't about to disappear. He had never quite been able to shake the sense of wistfulness, the *natsukashii* impression of lost sweetness, that had come over him as we had gone to repeat my blood tests a month before. This was not like John. His upbringing, so rich in the twin ethics of hard work and positive thinking, hadn't prepared him to wrap his mind around such delicate and unwelcome emotions. Years later, I would tell Katie that John and I got married so that he could teach me how to be happy and I could teach him how to be sad. She understood this immediately, as children always understand accurate assessments of their parents' emotional lives. John and I were both struggling, in our separate ways, to contain the strange rising tide of feelings. We would talk about it later; neither one of us mentioned it to the other when it was actually happening. This strikes me now as a terrible waste.

Of course, John had very little time for emotions of any kind. There was work to be done. A lot of work. An infinite amount of work. There is enough work at Harvard to bury a lifetime's worth of feelings, which is exactly what I think many of the university's residents are doing there. John got right back on the treadmill, if not eagerly, at least with a sense of familiarity. He was so used to the intense, constant pressure that the very discomfort of his Harvard lifestyle felt perversely comfortable.

Part of the reason John had so much to do was that he was compensating for my fragility and lack of energy. He urged me to do as little as possible and set out to accomplish everything necessary to care for all three of his dependents. Apart from his academic chores, he also shopped and cleaned and scheduled backup support for me during his future trips to Asia. Sibyl and Deirdre had already volunteered their services, and when they wouldn't be available, Katie and I would be flying to visit various family members who could care for us while John was out of the country. I protested all of this, feeling ashamed to require day care as much as Katie, but my concern for my unborn baby's health ultimately carried the vote, and I consented to John's elaborate plans.

Of course, John and I never told anyone connected to Harvard how close we were to cracking up. I still hadn't admitted to most of my acquaintances there that I was pregnant. By January, they all knew anyway. As I neared six months' gestation, my body blossomed into full-scale, unmistakable pregnancy. If you've ever been pregnant, you know how suddenly this happens. Within a couple of weeks my slight pot-gut became a prow to rival the *Queen Mary*'s. My abdomen preceded me into rooms and lurked heavily on my lap whenever I sat, so that I had to yank myself out of chairs. I took to wearing a large woolen overcoat that John had bought for himself at a secondhand store when we were undergraduates. It gave me a strong resemblance to Orson Welles in his later years. I was afraid that if I fainted on the street again, concerned bystanders would focus all their rescue efforts on pushing me back into the sea.

And so, as I waddled ever more slowly through the subzero temperatures and dirty gray light of that January, John dashed around Cambridge at accelerating speed, doing everything he could to keep our professional lives up and running. On one morning in particular, he had a great deal to do. He got up at dawn, fed and dressed Katie, made her lunch, and hoisted her into her backpack. Then he rushed over to Memorial Hall to register for classes. Next he proceeded to the day-care center, where he unpacked Katie and stayed for several hours, acting as the morning's parent volunteer. (In case there's any confusion here, this task was not voluntary. You could decide not to do it, but then your child would be expelled from the center and probably end up in some inferior day-care establishment, which would give her a serious disadvantage when it came to enrolling in the top kindergarten programs, which in turn would hurt her chances for admission at the best elementary, secondary, and high schools, and possibly, God forbid, scuttle her chances of getting into the Ivy League. I'm serious. This is really truly how parents we met through that day-care center talked as they picked up their children in the afternoons.)

When he was finished at the day-care center, John walked over to William James Hall. He was carrying two large cards with class listings on them, one for himself and one for me. The cards had to be signed by the appropriate professors before we could attend the classes we'd chosen. Harvard professors try to be accommodating during the first few days of the term, but they are inundated by students, and it isn't easy to track down all the right instructors and get their signatures. It took John the rest of that morning and half the afternoon to fill in most of the blanks on our registration cards. By 3:00 P.M. there was only one signature missing.

The necessary name belonged to an academician who had great power over John's educational career. This man was a legend in his field—revered at Harvard, recognizable even to lay readers of the more esoteric magazines. I'm not going to tell you his name, or his field, or exactly how he was related to John's academic progress, other than to say he was one of several people who would ultimately advise John on his dissertation. We will know him as Professor Goatstroke, because he wore a short white goatee, which he used to fondle a great deal, as though stroking a cat.

Professor Goatstroke was one of John's heroes, the closest thing he had to a mentor at Harvard. On the afternoon John was collecting registration-card signatures, the two had made an appointment to meet and discuss John's progress on his dissertation. To have a one-on-one appointment with Goatstroke, who spent a lot of his time with Nobel Prize winners and heads of state, was a tremendous—and tremendously high-pressured—honor.

John arrived a little early. Through the frosted glass door of Goatstroke's office, he could see the great scholar sitting at his desk, petting his beard as he read through a stack of articles. John paced nervously in the hall while he waited for the precise appointed time to knock on the door. He didn't want to stop moving. Every time he stopped moving, jet lag and sleep deprivation hit him like a board. Sleep had begun to sneak up on John at odd times and places; while he was waiting at a subway stop, talking on the phone, reading in the library. I would often come into our bedroom to find him sitting in front of his computer with not only his hands but also his face resting firmly on the keyboard. He staggered around our apartment wearing little computer-key indentations in his forehead, his dissertation progressing at something less than the speed of light. He was far behind the optimistic deadlines he and his advisers had set earlier in the academic year.

This meant that his visit to Professor Goatstroke's office that January day was fraught with even more than the usual tension. John took a deep breath before knocking on the great man's door, trying to raise his energy to its usual level, so that he could appear charming, articulate, and self-assured. It didn't work very well. He finally set himself the lofty goal of trying not to doze off during the meeting, and knocked.

Goatstroke's office was typical, for Harvard: a small, warm, cluttered room with a hardwood floor and a high ceiling. The rich smells of books and coffee washed over John as he went in. The view from the windows was partially obstructed by the leathery, maroon leaves of winter ivy. It may not have looked like much to an outsider, but we Harvard types knew that an office like this was the Olympic gold medal, the Oscar statuette of the academic world. Only the best of the best ever occupied one of them for an entire career. Walking into it, John felt like a child walking into a church.

"Oh, hello, John," said Goatstroke.

To have the scholar speak to him thus was, in itself, a notable distinction. John had taken classes from Goatstroke as an undergraduate, and the professor had usually addressed him as Mr. Beck. The formal address, though courteous, was not a mark of respect. It stressed the fact that Goatstroke and John were not peers. At John's graduation, as at every Harvard graduation for centuries, the president of the college closed the ceremony by saying to the new graduates, "I admit you to the society of educated men and women." (The "women" part, of course, was put in much later than the rest of it.) John and I both laughed at the self-congratulatory bombast of that little phrase. A few months later, however, after John had begun his doctoral work, we encountered Professor Goatstroke walking through Harvard Yard, and he said, "Hello, John." I swear John got visibly taller. It was like having Jesus pick him out of a crowd.

"Sit down, sit down," said Goatstroke cordially, waving toward a chair.

"Thanks," John said. He sat, hoping his body wouldn't take this as a signal to fall asleep.

"So, when did you get back from Asia?" Goatstroke smiled. He knew about John's consultancy work, and he wholeheartedly approved of it. The idea that one of his students was splitting his time between the Far East and Boston tickled him pink. He scratched his beard a little and then smoothed it carefully back into place.

"Uh, let's see," said John, doing his best to smile back. "I think it's been four days."

Goatstroke chuckled. "Amazing," he said. "When I first began studying Asia, it took ten days on a boat to get to Japan—and you didn't come home unless you had a damn good reason."

John shrugged amiably.

"So," said the professor. "Let's talk about the dissertation."

This created a tiny surge of adrenaline, as John prepared to confess that he was far behind on his production schedule. He had spent four hours at his computer the previous day, and written exactly three sentences worth keeping.

"I assume you've read Cantrell's latest work," said Goatstroke. He patted a book that lay open on his desk. "Groundbreaking stuff, don't you think? You'll have to address it."

"Right," said John. "Of course. Oh, I plan to."

Goatstroke looked at him knowingly. "What do you think of his arguments?" he asked casually. "What are the logical flaws?"

John blinked like an owl. "I plan to look at the book," he said, "but I haven't had a chance to read it carefully yet."

Goatstroke nodded, arching an eyebrow. John knew he had been tested and found lacking.

"So," said the older man, leaning back in his chair and grooming the little white beard with his fingertips, "exactly what *have* you had a chance to do?"

John took a deep breath, which made his head spin. "Well," he said, "I've done a lot of fieldwork on the ground in Tokyo. Not exactly the kind of stuff I can sum up until I have a chance to analyze it all."

He stopped and swallowed. Goatstroke was still looking at him, his fingers methodically massaging his facial hair. He hadn't even blinked.

"I don't think I'll have any trouble meeting my deadline," John lied. "It's just that the research is following a different course than I expected. I've basically just been putting all my ducks in a row, so to speak. Once that's done, you know how easy it is—you just knock them all over."

"I see," said Goatstroke heavily. "And when do you anticipate that this duck knocking will begin?"

It was all John could do not to squirm in his chair. The only thing that saved him was his complete lack of physical energy.

"I should be ready to start writing any day now," he said. "Of course, there are still a few loose ends in the field research. I'll tie those up on my next trip."

"You know, John," said Goatstroke, leaning forward and lacing his fingers together, "my colleagues and I are expecting sound work from you." He meant himself and John's other advisers, all of whom were chock full o' fame and prestige. "We admitted you to the program based on those expectations, and you can fulfill them—if you choose. You are capable of a great deal. It all depends on your decisions. How will you allocate your time? Your energy? Your thoughts?"

John nodded, dropping his eyes to Goatstroke's desk. He knew what his mentor had left unsaid. Many of John's professors had been unpleasantly surprised by the choices John made during his graduate school career, specifically, marrying me and fathering Katie. Goatstroke had often, though subtly, expressed his regret that John had chosen to dissipate his energy on "personal" issues at precisely the time when he could have been a rising star in his academic field.

Now, with Goatstroke's eyes boring into him, John knew that he should have followed his mentor's advice all along. He clamped his teeth a little tighter and told himself that it was time to get back on track. He had been weak. He had let himself forget his real priorities. But from that moment on, things were going to change. John would resolutely close his mind and heart to anything that would derail his work, pour himself into his research and writing as though nothing else existed.

John raised his eyes to meet Goatstroke's. "I'll have a chapter to you by Thursday," he said.

Goatstroke continued to look steadily at John for a moment. Then he smiled. His all-seeing eyes had discerned the switch in John's intentions, the firming of his resolve.

"Good," he said. "I'll look forward to seeing it."

There was little left to say. Goatstroke approved John's proposed course of study for the next semester and signed the registration card, they exchanged a few pleasantries, and John got up to go. His head was still swimming, but his will was strong. When he left the building and the blasting wind took his breath away, he welcomed it, opening his jacket so that the cold would keep him awake. It galvanized him to action. It reminded him who he really was, and what his priorities should be.

It was 3:30 P.M., already getting dark, as John rushed back to the day-care center to pick up Katie. He kissed her, as usual, before he strapped her onto his back, but after that he broke their usual routine. Most days, he would teach Katie colors by pointing out different cars along their route. This, however, was the beginning of John's new, more committed lifestyle. When Katie asked about the colors, he told her to hush and went back to thinking about his dissertation. That was the real problem, he told himself—not that he wasn't spending enough time writing but that he had let his *thoughts* stray from academic subjects. Colored cars, indeed. A successful man, a scholar, lived in his subject matter twenty-four hours a day. That was what John intended to do, from that day forward.

As he and Katie rode the apartment elevator up to the tenth floor, John rehearsed a little speech he was planning to give me, explaining that he simply couldn't afford to let his work slip any longer, that from now on he would not be spending time in rambling conversation or simple wordless companionship. Nothing, nothing, nothing would be allowed to distract him from his work. Otherwise, he would lose the prize he had been working for his entire life. John knew I wouldn't be happy about this, but I would understand. After all, I was Harvard too.

John opened the door firmly, with authority. He unpacked Katie, wiped the salt and grit off his heavy boots, and strode down the hall to the bedroom. In order to soften me up for his speech, he plastered a huge, sunshiny smile across his face.

The smile faded as soon as John saw me. I was standing in the middle of our bedroom, clutching the telephone receiver to my ear, with no color or expression on my face. I stared straight at John as though I hadn't seen him at all. Before I even spoke, before I even told him what had happened, the world John had so carefully constructed, the one he had resolved so desperately to preserve, began to fly apart in all directions. It would never be the same again.

21

➤ I propose that those of us who know the truth about telephones band together and form an association. We could call ourselves Phone Phobics Anonymous and hold conferences to discuss the many ways that telephones threaten public safety. We could commune about the way telephones make us feel; about the sick ambivalence that strikes us whenever a phone rings, about the way we sit and look at one, wondering what might happen to us if we pick it up. Veteran phone phobics such as myself could advise neophytes about strategies for refusing to answer the telephone at all, as well as basic self-defense techniques for those moments when their merciless attacks simply can't be avoided.

Here in Arizona, during the late-summer electric storms, the Powers That Be broadcast warnings advising people not to make telephone calls when it's raining. Lightning, they tell us, can travel through phone lines, right into your house, right into your ear. I once saw a man on television who had heard this bit of advice but was afraid his elderly mother hadn't. He called Mom during a storm to pass along the warning. Naturally (you saw this coming), while they were having the conversation a bolt of lightning zigged right into the man's phone line and up through the earpiece. Blasted the guy plum across the room, and now he can't conjugate verbs. That's what phones can do to you.

Of course, it would be a mistake to assume that telephones are innocuous except during stormy weather. No, no, no. They can deliver lightning bolts into your life on the sunniest of days. This is why we need our phone phobics association—to warn the unsuspecting. I wish someone had told me how much damage a telephone could do before that January day when the nurse-practitioner from University Health Services called me with the results of my amniocentesis.

It was another colorless, frozen afternoon in Cambridge. I was trying to get through some reading for one of my classes. I wasn't having much success. The books were incredibly dull, the kind of material you can't force yourself to absorb without entering some sort of sensory deprivation chamber, alone. This had become impossible for me—at five and a half months' gestation, I had company wherever I went. Adam was now fully formed enough to do all sorts of calisthenics but not yet so big that his movements were cramped by the limited rental space in my abdomen. It had become disgracefully easy for him to tempt me into coming out to play.

We had a little game we liked a lot. I called it Prod. We didn't play much when I was up and around, because the motion of my body tended to lull Adam to sleep. But when I sat still he'd wake up and thump on the walls to tell me he was there. I'd be reading along, trying to focus on something like statistical evidence of long-term economic depression among pink-collar workers in southwestern Detroit, when suddenly I'd feel a firm poke from my insides. I could rarely resist pulling my sweater tight around my belly and watching in amazement as the small, rather pointy shape of a hand or foot bulged outward from my own body. I would push on the protrusion with my hand and feel the baby float in the opposite direction, until he bumped against my spine or something and rebounded outward. Then he'd prod me again and we'd repeat the whole procedure.

We could play for hours.

This was what I was doing that day when the telephone rang. I was enjoying Prod so much that it never even occurred to me to be afraid. I was young and naive; I just slapped the receiver to my ear and said hello.

"Hello, Martha?"

"Speaking." I recognized the voice.

"It's Judy Trenton," she said. "From University Health Services."

"Right," I said. "Hi, Judy."

I was pleased that she had called me by my first name. Most of the clinic personnel called me Mrs. Beck, which made me feel like an aged hausfrau. I now understand that Judy's first-name familiarity was a danger signal, a clear sign that I should slam down the telephone receiver and run away fast.

"I have some . . . not so good news for you," said Judy. She sounded strange. Robotic. "The results from your amniocentesis are in, and they show that you are carrying a Down syndrome fetus."

I didn't say anything. I felt as though I were falling through space. What I remember most about that moment are the details of the room: the maroon quilt on the futon, the clutter of papers on the desk, the smoke smudges on the walls. The smudges had been there ever since Food Shak burned. No matter how we scrubbed at them, they wouldn't come off.

"Martha?" Judy Trenton's voice wasn't so dispassionate anymore. Now she sounded a little frightened.

"Oh, my God," I said. I sat down slowly on the futon. The room began to turn hazy. I pulled my feet onto the futon and curled my head down between my knees so that I wouldn't faint.

"Martha? Martha, are you there?"

"I'm here," I whispered.

Judy said something else. I don't remember what. I didn't hear her, because there was someone else speaking to me at the same time—or perhaps I should say some*thing*.

The voice was very clear. It didn't come through my ears; it simply appeared inside my mind like dew appearing on flowers at dawn. You couldn't say exactly where it came from, but there it was.

Don't be afraid.

Those were the only words. But words were just a tiny fraction of the message. From the warmth of the voice, from its incredible gentleness, I knew that "Don't be afraid" was not a commandment to be brave, not a dismissal of my fear, not a testament to the power of positive thinking. It simply meant that there was nothing to fear in the first place. It meant that I was safe. That it would never let anything hurt me.

The comfort that voice brought with it flickered out in a heartbeat. Then the apartment zoomed into focus around me, and I was sitting in a cold room, alone, with my world turned upside down.

"Martha? Martha? *Martha?*"

"Yeah."

Judy's voice had lost its mechanical timbre. Now she sounded almost desperate. "Do you still feel the same way about . . . about not terminating the pregnancy?" she said. "There's still time if you want to change your mind. Not much, but there is still time."

I took a long breath. Everything I had ever striven for, every hope I'd ever hoped and dream I'd ever dreamt, seemed to be poised like a delicate Fabergé egg between the tips of my fingers.

"No," I whispered. The egg fell, smashing into a million shards on the floor.

I want you to know that this was not a decision made out of ethical principles. I was going on sheer emotion. If I had been one of those women whose pregnancies progress smoothly and easily, I might very well have chosen an abortion. But I had struggled so hard and endured so much already, trying to keep Adam alive, that I had built up tremendous momentum in that direction. By the time the Down syndrome was diagnosed, I could no more have asked for an abortion than I could have shot Katie in the head.

"No," I repeated to Judy, "I don't want to terminate the pregnancy."

"I see." Judy sounded absolutely miserable. I knew she was trying as hard as she could not to second-guess my decision. "I'm sorry," she said at last.

"Thanks."

"Is there anything I could help you with?" she said. "Do you have any questions?"

I closed my eyes. Of course I had questions. I had nothing but questions.

"I guess . . . I mean, I've heard . . ." My voice faltered and went silent.

"Yes?" said Judy.

"I've heard that people with Down syndrome can be . . ." I groped for the right word. "I've heard they can be . . . happy."

That is right.

It was such a calm voice, so completely without judgment or condemnation. I felt absolutely certain that if I had chosen to have an abortion, the owner of that voice would have loved and approved of me every bit as much.

Judy paused for a minute. "I guess they can be happy," she said at last. "I don't really know."

I appreciated her honesty. At times like that, when you are stripped down to an intolerable reality, glib reassurances stink of falsehood. Trust me; I've heard plenty.

"I've been . . . I've been looking things up," said Judy. "About Down syndrome. The fetus you're carrying is a typical trisomy-twenty-one."

I was still curled into a ball on the futon, the phone receiver crushed to my ear. "What does that mean?" I said.

"It means that at conception, one of the haploid cells, either the egg or the sperm, failed to fully divide before fertilization. Then, when the cells combine, you get three chromosomes in the twenty-first position instead of two. The fetus has forty-seven chromosomes, instead of forty-six, and—"

"I know that!" I barked the words into the phone, not caring how rude I was being. "I've taken biology, for God's sake! I said what does it *mean*?"

There was a pause. Then Judy said, "I'm not sure I understand."

"What does it mean to my life—to our lives?" I said. "What's going to happen?"

"I don't know." Judy sounded very sad. I myself felt no emotion at all, only that dreadful falling sensation.

"Well," said Judy, "I guess that's all there is to say. Listen, Martha, if you have any questions, I'm always—"

"Don't hang up!" I said desperately, ashamed by the open neediness in my voice. "Please, don't hang up!"

"Okay, okay," she said. "I'm still here. Martha, is your husband home?"

"No, he's . . . he'll be home . . ." I couldn't organize my thoughts at all. "We were going to put the baby in the day-care center—we already reserved a slot in the newborn room. Now I guess that won't happen."

"No," said Judy.

"We won't even be able to get anyone to baby-sit," I said.

"Maybe not." Judy Trenton had the instincts of a true healer—she was kind, but even more important, she was honest. She was also dead wrong. But neither of us knew that at the time.

My mind was racing through that mass of questions like a ricocheting bullet. I tried to focus on one at a time, to say something—anything—that would keep Judy from hanging up and leaving me by myself with a deformed baby.

"How do you know?" I said, almost to myself.

"Know what?" Judy asked softly.

"How do you know who should live? Is it such a bad thing not to live?"

Judy said nothing. She seemed to know that listening was more important.

"I used to think a lot about suicide," I said. During my teenage existential crisis, I had thought that knowing the Meaning of Life was an abstract, esoteric question. Now I felt that it was an absolute necessity.

"Martha, please!" Judy cried. "Don't talk that way—we have a psychologist here, I could refer you—"

"No, no, no," I snapped. "I'm not going to kill myself *now*, for crying out loud. That was a long time ago, when I was trying to figure out the meaning of life, and I read all this philosophy, and—but you know what, Judy? They didn't really understand. Not any of them. Not Plato, not Kant, not any of the big boys."

I was aware, in a distant way, that I was talking like the schizophrenic homeless people who prowled the streets of Cambridge. There was one old woman with a toupee who slept in the Science Center at night, leaning against her brown paper bag. The first year I was at Harvard, one of my fellow freshmen sneaked a peek inside that bag at about 2:00 A.M. on a sleepless night and discovered that it held—more bags. I knew I resembled that old woman as I babbled to Judy on the telephone, but I couldn't seem to stop.

"None of those philosophers got the point," I told her.

"Oh?" Judy's voice was uncertain. One can hardly blame her.

"No," I said. "Because they were always focusing on what happens to people. The meaning of life is not what happens to people."

"It's not?"

"No, it's not," I said. "The meaning of life is what happens *between* people."

"I see," said Judy, though I wasn't really sure she did.

The next thing I said was, "What?" But I wasn't even talking to Judy. I was talking to the other voice, the voice inside my head, the voice inside my heart. This time, it asked me a question.

Martha, are you happy?

"Happy?" I repeated. It seemed like a strange question to me. I was used to thinking in terms of whether or not I was successful, accepted, noteworthy. It had been a long time since I had even thought about being happy.

"Martha?" said Judy gingerly, no doubt convinced that the bad news had driven me right over the edge of the cracker barrel. "Martha, are you all right?"

"Yes, I'm all right, I'm all right," I said. I was still thinking about happiness. I had just realized that I didn't have a clue what it was.

Then Adam kicked me in the ribs. It was one of his "Come out and play!" kicks; he wanted me to join him in a game of Prod. I felt a gush of absolute horror, a mixture of grief and fear so strong it almost knocked me out. I wrapped my free hand—the one not holding the phone—around my knees, so that my body formed a tight little ball around Adam's playroom. Then I began to rock slightly, back and forth, back and forth, back and forth. It helped.

Judy Trenton had been talking into the phone for about a minute, getting no response from me. Finally she said, "Listen, Martha, how close are you to Harvard Square?"

"Pretty close," I said, rocking. "Pretty close."

"Why don't you come in?" said Judy. "My last appointment is at four. Can you make it at four-thirty?"

"Okay," I gasped. I had finally begun to cry, but it was a weak, tepid sort of cry, not nearly big enough for the emotions I had to process. The rocking numbed me, pushed the horror into a kind of holding zone at the back of my soul. It was like buying pain on credit.

"I'm sorry, Judy," I said.

"What?" She sounded confused. "*You're* sorry?"

"I'm sorry you had to make a call like this. It must be awful."

Long pause.

"It is." Now Judy was crying too. "I'd like to give you a hug."

Then I realized that she understood after all. About the Meaning of Life.

There was a thump in the hallway outside our apartment door; the sound of the elevator arriving at our floor. Then the jangle and click of John's key in the lock.

"Judy!" I whispered, almost panicking. "John's here!"

"Oh, good." Her voice was heavy with relief.

I stood up, the blood rushing from my head and making me teeter before I got my feet solidly under me.

"I have to tell him," I said. "I have to tell him."

John's voice, dreadfully tired and hoarse but resolutely cheerful, came from the living room. "Hi, Marth! We're back!"

꜋ I tried to pull myself together before he opened the bedroom door. I tried to put on some kind of smile, to greet him warmly, to give him a moment of peace before he had to know. But as soon as John saw my face, before I said a word, I could tell it was too late for that.

"Good-bye, Judy," I whispered into the mouthpiece, my eyes locked on John's. "Thanks."

Then I hung up the telephone, that terrible, terrible instrument of destruction. The phone just sat there, as if it hadn't done anything bad at all.

22

✎ Every December my friend Annette, who in other respects is a very nice person, spends an inordinate amount of time and money obtaining the most obnoxious toy gun on the market for Adam's Christmas present. I don't give my children guns as toys, but as Adam's honorary auntie, Annette feels that it is her right and responsibility to indulge the kid's most violent, macho, antisocial tendencies.

Adam loves her very much.

Annette's first criterion, when purchasing the Christmas gun, is wattage. She looks for a product that makes enough noise to disrupt the breeding process for every bird living within a mile radius of our house. Flashing lights rank a close second. Annette prefers guns that flash several colors, all bright enough to stun the average person's retina, so that for a couple of minutes after Adam fires the gun at you, you walk blindly into walls and pillars and closed glass doors. It is also very important to have an innovative design, with various exotic flanges meant to suggest deadliness of interplanetary proportions.

It goes without saying that guns of this magnitude require dozens of large batteries. Annette never forgets this; she always buys an ample supply of them, wrapping them in a separate package, which she tapes to the actual gun. I'm telling you, the woman has absolutely no mercy.

The first Christmas after Annette and I got to know each other, my children arose at a predictably ungodly hour and descended on their gifts like locusts on an alfalfa field. Along with most other American parents, John and I had spent a good part of the previous month tracking down the items our children had requested in their letters to Santa. Katie had asked for a set of birdcalls she'd seen in an FAO Schwarz catalog. Five-year-old Lizzie wanted one of those dolls they advertise on Saturday morning cartoons, the ones that have repulsively cute names and have been engineered to mimic the least pleasant behaviors of real human babies. I think that year Lizzie's doll had an anxiety-related bed-wetting disorder or something. Adam wanted a whole brigade of toys with names like Cretin Slime Monsters.

In the proud tradition of delayed gratification John inherited from a long line of Becks, the children opened their presents one by one. Katie went first. The FAO Schwarz birdcall set had turned out to cost several hundred dollars, so John and I had purchased what we thought was a reasonable facsimile. It didn't cover quite as broad an ornithological spectrum as the pricier set, but it could produce a great duck sound, a good owl, and several very convincing songbirds. When she saw it, Katie's face fell. It is an awful thing to see your kid's face fall on Christmas morning.

"Don't you like it?" I asked anxiously.

"No, no, it's okay. I like it." Katie smiled a stalwart smile, but her lower lip trembled ever so slightly. I began to feel that perhaps we should have taken out a second mortgage to pay for the FAO Schwarz birdcall set.

Lizzie went next. She tore the gift wrapping off her bed-wetting doll, and then she, too, developed that troubled look around the eyes.

"What's the matter?" I asked.

"Well," said Lizzie, with her high voice and precocious vocabulary, "it's not exactly what I asked for."

John, who had fought his way through about seventeen toy stores looking for that particular doll, burst out, "I thought you *wanted* a Tiny Whiny Princess Wee-Wee!"

"I did," said Lizzie, "but I wanted the one with the *pink* jewels, and this one only has the *purple* jewels."

Within minutes, both the girls had reconciled themselves to their gifts. Like their pioneer ancestors, many of whom had died crossing the Great Plains on foot in the dead of winter, dragging their possessions behind them in handcarts, my daughters were able to steel themselves to the brutal realities of an imperfect world. This was good, because I had been on the verge of sending them both to military school.

Now it was Adam's turn. He fished around under the Christmas tree until he found a package with his name on it. It was from Annette. He tore the paper off, holding his breath, and found—batteries. An eight-pack of double D's, still encased in plastic.

"Oh, honey," I said, "that's not the real present. The real present is—"

But Adam didn't hear me. He was staring at those batteries as if they were so magnificent he couldn't quite take them in. His mouth fell open in astonished ecstasy as he held the batteries up to the light.

"Oh, wow!" he said. "*Oh, wow!* Mom, look! *Batteries!*" (It actually sounded more like "Mom, ook! *Aggabies!*" but the message was clear.)

Before we could divert his attention to any other gift, Adam leapt to his feet and began running around the house, locating every appliance, tool, and toy that ran on batteries. The whole time, he babbled excitedly about all the things he could do with this fabulous, fabulous gift. As we watched, it began to occur to all of us "normal" people in the family that batteries really were a pretty darn good Christmas present. They didn't look like much, on the face of it, but think what they could *do*! Put them in place, and inanimate objects suddenly came to life, moving, talking, singing, lighting up the room. Something about Adam always manages to see straight past the outward ordinariness of a thing to any magic it may hold inside. We wouldn't even have bothered to let him open the gun, except that we were afraid Annette would buy him a neutron bomb for his birthday if we didn't.

I bring this up because, looking back on the journal I kept while I was expecting Adam, I find that before he was even born, I was already comparing him to a disappointing holiday gift. I must mention that this journal was not meant to be read by others. It was the secret place where I poured out my most distasteful and shocking emotions, to keep myself from going insane during the endless, frightening months between his diagnosis and his birth.

"Last week," I wrote one January afternoon, "a homeless man I passed in Harvard Square took one look at my belly and said, 'Congratulations, Mamma!' I've almost forgotten what it was like to have people react that way. Nobody does, since we found out about the Down syndrome. The baby has become unmentionable, like a gift everyone knows is inferior and broken, before it's even unwrapped."

This comment was largely true, although perhaps a bit too absolute. Not "everyone" stopped treating me like a pregnant woman and began acting as if I'd contracted a terminal illness. But precious few of the exceptions came from within the Harvard community, the community that had been my reference group, my "ideal" culture, since I was seventeen years old. No one at Harvard seemed able to tolerate the thought of Santa's leaving the wrong kind of baby under the tree. It was very clear what kind of children most Harvard types would have asked for in their letters to Santa. I realized this not much more than an hour after I learned about Adam's Down syndrome.

I left the apartment soon after John came home. In our marriage, the unspoken rule had always been that when one of us was upset, the other would compensate by being strong and encouraging. We'd switch roles after the upset person began to feel a little better. It reminded me of mountaineering teams whose members take turns scaling unconquered territory, planting ropes on a vertical rock face and then helping their partners up a few feet. The day we found out about Adam strained this system to its breaking point. I was far too devastated to comfort John. Perhaps if he'd been any less tired or jet-lagged or worried about school, he could have soldiered through and comforted me. But he was already carrying a heavy burden, and the news that one's unborn son is going to be mentally retarded isn't merely a straw to break the camel's back. It's more like a sack of headstones.

It's painful to remember the way John's face looked when I told him; so painful that I can barely summon the memory. He went very, very pale. Then he came slowly over, as though he were sleepwalking, and put his arms around me. He was as cold as a statue.

"You're going to keep him, aren't you?" he said.

I nodded slowly, my face against his chest.

"So that's why," said John. "So that's why."

I looked up at him. "What do you mean?"

John was staring over my head at the window. The light that came through it was dim and gray.

"In the restaurant, that day," he said. "The day you got the tests done. Do you remember?"

I nodded again.

"We were sitting there, and you were talking about abortion, and then . . ." John's voice trailed off and he shook his head. "It was probably just my imagination. But it was so—so *strong*."

I felt a prickle of electricity go up my spine. I pulled back my head and looked up into his haggard, beloved face. "What was so strong?"

He closed his eyes and swallowed. Then he said, very reluctantly, "I heard this . . . voice."

I said nothing. I had known what he was going to tell me before he said it.

John continued even more slowly. "It said something."

I knew exactly what he was feeling, exactly why it seemed physically painful for him to tell me. He was fighting through the same walls of disbelief, the same fear of ridicule, the same shame I felt when I thought of talking to anyone about the inexplicable things that had happened to me. He didn't know about the decision I had made—to believe anything, everything, until it was proven false—and I was too stunned to explain.

I just asked, "What did it say?"

John shook his head, as though to apologize for what he was about to tell me. "It said, '*John, keep the baby.*'" John looked down at me, and his face suddenly looked concerned. "I mean, I know it isn't my decision, it's *your* decision, but—"

I set one finger on his lips. "It's okay," I said, although of course nothing was okay.

"The thing is," said John, "it wasn't like an order. It felt more like someone was giving me advice, someone who knew more than I did." He bit his lip hard, and I could see that the memory made him want to cry. "It sounded very kind," he concluded.

"I know," I said.

"Do you think I'm crazy?" John sounded like a little boy.

I shook my head. "Look what I'm doing," I said. I put a hand on my swollen midsection. "Do you think *I'm* crazy?"

He shook his head but said nothing. We were both too overwhelmed to talk anymore. I didn't know how to begin telling John about the Bunraku puppeteers, about the strange things I had experienced during the last five months. I was somewhat surprised and slightly comforted to know that John, too, had heard one of the voices, and I was immensely relieved that the experience seemed to have discouraged him from pressuring me to abort the baby. But what might have intrigued and excited me in different circumstances barely seemed worth thinking about now that I was trying to adjust to being the mother of a retarded child.

John and I stood there in silence for several minutes, until it was clear that neither one of us was prepared to be the strong one, to take the lead on this particular mountaineering expedition. We had reached a spot beyond our ability to cope as a team. So without another word, we disengaged, and each of us reverted to the behaviors we had used to cope with disturbing information for most of our lives.

For John, this meant a ferocious concentration on work. He went into a frenzy of activity, typing up notes for his dissertation, giving Katie her dinner, making phone calls to Singapore, doing the laundry. The movement of his mind and muscles, the simplicity and solidness of work, seemed to allow him to shut down his awareness of what was happening to his personal life. He was a Harvard kind of guy.

To me, John's behavior was incomprehensible. I couldn't focus on anything but my fear and grief. My way of coping with this situation—with any situation—was to learn everything I could about it, to follow my credo that knowledge is power. Knowledge had helped me dull the pain and fear of being different ever since I had learned how to talk. And so, before I even stopped at Judy Trenton's office on that day she called with the "not so good news," I made for the bookstore section of the Harvard Coop to look for information about raising a child with Down syndrome.

The Coop is Harvard's official bookstore, the one that stocks all the textbooks and required readings for classes. It sells everything from Harvard insignia T-shirts to snack foods, and it has one of the largest and best-equipped book sections of any college store in the country. I had never spent much time browsing the "parenting" section. Before Katie was born, I had a hard time believing that an actual baby was going to come out of me, let alone survive the event. After her birth, I was busy forcing myself through thousands of pages of required sociological theory—this at a time when I was too tired to really focus on anything longer than a haiku. I never got around to reading much about how to raise children, not even an article in *Woman's Day.* I decided that feeling guilty about *not* reading such things would have to be good enough.

At least I knew which section of the Coop contained books on parenting. I lugged my abdomen toward Harvard Square, keeping my eyes fixed on the cobblestones directly in front of me. This was how I kept myself from coming apart. I had never meditated before, but over the next few months I would figure out how to do it without any instruction at all. I learned to wash my mind blank and stare at some object, real or imagined, until I felt as though I were floating in a state of being that was nearly, but not precisely, alive. I devised mantras, phrases I repeated over and over to help me stop thinking. I remember vividly the mantra that got me from my apartment to the Coop that afternoon. As I walked along the slushy sidewalks under a freezing rain, I murmured over and over, "Why not me? Why not me? Why not me?"

I can honestly say I never did ask the opposite question. The answer seemed obvious. I have been the beneficiary of so much improbable good fortune in my life that it's only logical I'd have some bad luck as well. What I did ask myself that day, what I continue to ask myself as I watch Adam go out into a frightening world in all his gentleness, sweetness, and hope, is, "Why him? Why him? Why him?" The hardest lesson I have ever had to learn is that I will never know the meaning of my children's pain, and that I have neither the capacity nor the right to take it away from them.

It was the thought of Adam's pain that finally broke through my numbness and let the full weight of my emotion bear down on me. Even though I loved my unborn baby with unreasoning intensity, I was terribly afraid for him. I was also terribly afraid *of* him. The bulge of my torso now seemed freakish, monstrous, grotesque. The baby inside it was broken. He was substandard. He was not what I had wanted.

Once I got to the Coop and made my way to the parenting section, I found a lot of examples of what I *had* wanted laid out in front of me. Four or five long bookshelves were occupied by instructional variations on a single subject: how to turn a human infant into a genius in the shortest time possible. The object, apparently, was to have every child— no, I'm sorry, make that "*your* child"—contributing important innovations to science and letters before it achieved bowel control. There were books recommending different shapes to hang from mobiles, thus stimulating your infant's intellectual development. There were sets of flash cards designed to help your tiny scholar's mind associate phonetic symbols with the appropriate sounds. Others promoted development across the whole behavioral spectrum, teaching everything from ethics to "killer competitiveness." I have seen many of these same books in other bookstores at other times, but only the Harvard Coop had *all* of them: *Teach Your Baby to Read; Born to Win; Pre-Law for Preschoolers; Toddling Through the Calculus.*

Staring at these titles through tear-glazed eyes, I felt like a kid holding a lump of coal, watching everyone else open gorgeous, desirable Tiny Whiny Princess Wee-Wees with the pink *and* purple jewels. For the first time in my life, I began to question why there should be so much material to help parents enhance their children's "excellence." Slowly, slowly, standing in the Coop, I realized that I was not looking for information to transform my child into a prize every parent would envy. I needed to transform *myself* into a parent who could accept her child, no matter what. There were no books for that in the parenting section of the Harvard Coop.

I left the parenting section without buying anything and proceeded up the escalator to the textbook section. There, after a half hour's search through the textbooks for abnormal psychology classes, I found a small book on how to train and teach the mentally retarded. The book was a mustard-yellow paperback with a photograph of two children on the cover. They both had Down syndrome. The picture was grainy and out of focus; the two children, lumpish and awkward-looking, stared dully at the camera through small, misshapen eyes. I cannot tell you how much it hurt me to look at that picture. It was like getting my heart caught in a mill saw.

I turned the book facedown and carried it to the cash register, focusing on the grimy linoleum floor tiles to keep my mind in suspended animation. Why not me? Why not me? Why not me? The woman at the cash register flipped the book over, and I saw the picture again. I almost ran for the door. I forced myself to look at the book's cover again as I handed over my money. Those two children in the picture were everything I had ever learned to avoid. Beneath a thin facade of polite pity, I found in myself a roiling sea of fear and loathing. The words that sprang to my mind as I looked at that picture were bluntly cruel. Stupid. Retard. Imbecile. Fool. Moron. Before that day, I would never have admitted, even to myself, that I ever thought such words about actual people. Now I was thinking them about a being who was not yet separate from me. *I* was a child on the cover of that book, and the horror of it was almost more than I could bear.

I finished paying for the book and rushed into the small elevator that went from the third-floor textbook section to ground level. The elevator was barely big enough for two slender people, and in my condition I pretty much filled it. I waited until it was between floors, then hit the stop button with a closed fist. I hit it much harder than necessary. Then I leaned back against the wall and covered my face with my hands, trying to control myself. I felt as though some evil ogre had killed my "real" baby—the baby I'd been expecting—and replaced him with an ugly, broken replica. My grief at losing that "real" baby was as intense as if he had been two years old, or five, or ten. The whole thing seemed wildly unfair to me: my baby was dead, and I was still pregnant. I was suddenly seized by a rage so strong I wanted to bash in the elevator walls.

Somewhere above the anger, my intellect registered all of this, reviewing the emotional stages of accepting a loss. First there was denial, I knew, then grief, then anger, then bargaining—no, wait, it was bargaining, then grief, then anger—or maybe anger, then bargaining, then grief? It felt as though all of them were assaulting me at once. I remembered that the final stage was acceptance. But then again, that was when the tragedy was a death. What if it wasn't? What if the tragedy was born alive? I tried to force myself to reach acceptance immediately, right there in the elevator, without wading into the morass of pain I could sense just ahead of me. I considered abortion again, but the pain that lay in that direction was even greater. It was easier for me—not better, mind you, not braver or nobler or morally superior, but *easier*—to have the baby. I wondered why the psychological stages of loss didn't include fear. Maybe it was because fear pervades and overwhelms everything else. I mashed my hands against my eyes and shook so hard that the elevator compartment trembled on its cable.

From here, ten years in the future, it seems ironically fitting that I locked myself, alone, into a cramped, cold, hard, barren space near the Coop's textbook section before I let myself feel my deep emotional reaction to Adam's diagnosis. For a few of my Harvard years, I taught drawing to architecture students, and during that time I became convinced that we human beings gravitate toward spaces that are metaphors for our inner lives. That elevator pretty much summed up the way I had learned to exist. I went into it in order to gain control, an effort that had consumed me for years. It worked fairly well. After only a few seconds, before anyone could hear the alarm and come to help, I punched the button again and proceeded to the ground floor. By the time the door slid open, I had stopped crying. I would not lose control of myself in public again for some time—definitely not when I went to see Judy Trenton, to find out just how many things were likely to be wrong with the unseen person I carried under my heart.

It was between the Coop and the clinic that I passed the homeless man who looked at my abdomen and said, "Congratulations, Mamma!" I glanced around, not realizing at first that he had been talking to me. I had already stopped believing that my pregnancy merited congratulations. If that man only knew, I thought bitterly. Now the memory makes me smile. I like to think that the homeless man may have been acting under the influence of the Bunraku puppeteers. Maybe he was one of them. I have a hunch that if he had known everything about my retarded baby, he would have congratulated me just as warmly. In my mind, I picture him showing the same astonished delight I saw in Adam on the Christmas morning when he unwrapped his batteries. This little boy may not look like what you asked for, the man might have told me. He may not have the features you requested, or be able to perform all the tricks. But put him in place, and he will light up your life. You have no idea how much magic is in him.

23

⤳ You can tell a great deal about people by the way they react when you tell them you're going to have a retarded child. You might want to try this on a few of your own friends, as a kind of litmus test to see what the world looks like to them. Of course, a lot depends on their personal histories—whether they have ever interacted with disabled people and what that interaction was like. But when you control for that factor (as we sociologists like to say), a person's reaction to the news of retardation is usually a distilled manifestation of his or her view of the universe.

Within a few hours of hearing Adam's diagnosis, John and I had called several of our friends and relations, looking for comfort. Instead, we found that we had bumbled into a place so alien and unfamiliar that virtually no one we spoke to had a clue as to what to say or do. My parents reacted as well as they could, but though unquestioningly supportive, they were almost as distressed as I was. My mother had always taken great pride in pointing out that she had borne eight healthy babies, all with high IQs (as frequently measured by our student neighbors). The concept of a retarded grandson stunned her to near silence. My father was so upset that he didn't even pick up the phone. My strongest feeling as I hung up was guilt at having brought this catastrophe into their lives.

John called his parents right after I called mine. I sat near him on the couch, my eyelids swollen and stinging with tears, and listened to his end of the conversation.

"Hi, Mom and Dad," said John. "How are you?"

Pause.

"That's good. Well, I'm all right, I guess. We just found out that the baby has Down syndrome. The new baby."

Pause.

"Down syndrome. I think they used to call it mongoloidism."

Pause.

"Um . . . Delta. I flew in on Delta last time."

Pause.

"I had chicken. It was pretty good. A little too well done."

John's parents went on asking him about airplane travel for ten minutes, and he kept responding politely, in a voice that sounded as though the blood had been drained from it. Finally, John's mother said, "Well, just be grateful you've got Katie." Then they hung up.

I was floored by the apparent indifference of this conversation, but John assured me that his parents were just trying to absorb the information. Sure enough, half an hour later they called back with words of support and sympathy. But the first go-round had shown me that Faye and Jay were as lost in this new obstetrical terrain as my own parents. It seemed utterly impossible that John and I could find our way back to a normal life.

I didn't sleep that night. I lay on the futon and stared at the ceiling, as numb as if I had been breathing nothing but airplane glue for weeks. John rolled and thrashed fitfully beside me, mumbling dark, meaningless syllables into his pillow. When we moved away from Cambridge, after Adam was born, we left that lumpy futon behind. It was the scene of more sickness and sadness than we cared to remember. We didn't even call it a mattress—we referred to it as a "stress mat." We hoped that its new owners would never know how dangerous it could be.

The next morning I was scheduled to have breakfast with Deirdre Hennesy and Sibyl Johnston. Deirdre picked me up right on time, looking as luminous as ever, with only a tidy little bulge below the navel to reveal her own pregnancy. We briefly discussed the best way to get to the little café where we were meeting Sibyl. I thought about trying to keep Adam's condition a secret. I thought about my parents' reaction, and my in-laws', and wondered if I could handle Deirdre's response should I decide to tell her. In the end, I simply couldn't hold it in. As she put the car in gear, I blurted, "My baby has Down syndrome."

Deirdre moved the gearshift back to park. Without a word, she leaned over and put her arms around my shoulders. My eyes filled with tears and I looked down quickly to hide them. Deirdre bowed her own head until her forehead rested against mine. I don't remember her saying anything. There was no need for it. I could feel her compassion, but what struck me more was her complete lack of fear or awkwardness. An amazing calm emanated from her to me. It was utterly different from the panic I had sensed from John's parents, and mine. I knew this was partly because Deirdre was more distant from the baby than our families, and she therefore had less to fear from his disabilities. But I believe the strength she was able to give me came from more than just that. I thought about Deirdre's story, about the old woman who had washed her when she was weak and defeated and ready to die. I felt grateful to the soles of my feet for that old woman's gift, a gift that was now being passed on to me.

Eventually we both straightened up again, and Deirdre drove to the café where we were meeting Sibyl. It was a cozy place with only a few tables. Half of it was occupied by a glass display case containing fresh baked goods. They smelled exquisite. I ordered a cranberry muffin. It looked and tasted delicious, but I couldn't swallow any of it. I might as well have tried to eat a lump of adobe.

Deirdre and I were sipping herbal tea when Sibyl pushed open the door and entered in a swirl of snow.

"Sorry I'm late," she said breathlessly. "Charles just got back from class to take Mie." She smiled. Deirdre and I did not. Sibyl's face went sober. "What's wrong?"

I had asked Deirdre to let me deliver the news myself. "My baby," I said. "Down syndrome."

Sibyl sat down slowly, forgetting to take off her coat. Snowflakes melted into tiny bright beads on her coppery hair.

"Oh, Martha."

I shrugged.

"Has the shock worn off yet?" she asked.

I shrugged again.

"It will," she said. "It may take a year or so until you feel normal again, but you're probably going through the worst of it right now."

There was so much confidence in her low, soothing voice that I felt something shift inside me, as though she had just wedged her own shoulder under the burden I was carrying.

"Have they put you in touch with anyone?" asked Sibyl. "Parent to Parent? The ARC?"

I squinted at her. "The what?"

"The Association for Retarded Citizens," she said. She dug through her purse. "Here, I'll give you their number."

Deirdre and I were both watching her incredulously. Deirdre said, "You have the number for the ARC in your *purse*?"

Sibyl nodded. "Here it is." She wrote on a scrap of paper from her planning calendar and pushed it across the small tabletop to me. Deirdre and I just sat and looked at her.

"What?" said Sibyl. "What are you guys staring at?"

I took the paper scrap off the table and held it up between my thumb and forefinger.

"Why?" I said.

Deirdre nodded.

Sibyl's porcelain skin flushed pink. "My book," she said.

I knew that Sibyl was a writer, that she spent hours every day in her home office working on her latest novel. But she had always been reluctant to talk about the book's content. We sometimes discussed her writing, but never the actual story she was telling. She didn't want to dissipate her energy in conversation, and I respected that.

Now Sibyl took a deep breath. "A few years ago, I got interested in a baby with a genetic defect," she said. "That's what my book is about."

"Down syndrome?" Deirdre asked her.

"No." Sibyl shook her head. "Worse." I noticed that it comforted me to remember there were worse genetic defects than Down syndrome. My reaction made me feel slightly guilty; it was awfully close to rejoicing in the bad fortune of others.

The waiter showed up, and Sibyl ordered her own herbal tea. Then she launched into a description of the research she had been doing for the past several years. It turned out that Sibyl was an absolute encyclopedia of information about having and raising a child with a disability.

She was a very thorough researcher, and she had a mind like flypaper— everything stuck to it. Even though the baby portrayed in her book didn't have Down syndrome, Sibyl knew the number of babies born with the condition every year; the percentage of those babies who had heart-valve defects, seizures, and harelips; the organizations set up to assist parents; and the latest advances in "early intervention" to help disabled children maximize their functional potential.

As I listened to Sibyl, I was once again overcome by the strange, electric feeling that had become so familiar to me during the past months. It was the same thing I had felt the first time Sibyl knocked on my apartment door, on the day when I was losing my fight with the nausea. Whoever or whatever had sent her to my aid that day undoubtedly knew that she brought more than groceries along with her. She also carried even more information and understanding about my baby than I could have gotten from the obstetrical specialists at University Health Services. The electric sensation tingled across my scalp until I expected to hear my individual hairs crackling against my ears like tiny power cables. *This is not accidental,* the feeling said. *None of it is an accident. You are not falling into nothing. Trust us. We will catch you. You have never been alone.*

⌒   In the meantime, on the other side of Cambridge, John was trying out the bad news on someone else, with rather less gratifying results. He was scheduled to meet with Professor Goatstroke again to review his progress. Although he had managed to hammer out a few pages of his dissertation the day before, the combination of a raging sore throat and the news about Adam had made it almost impossible for him to concentrate. The chapter wasn't finished, and what he had wasn't top quality. John's pounding head filled with foreboding as he knocked on Goatstroke's office door.

"Come in," said the professor.

John opened the door. Goatstroke was reading an academic journal. He gestured toward the wooden chair that faced his desk. John sat down silently and looked around the room, waiting for his mentor to finish. The coffeemaker was perking away on the filing cabinet. The steam that rose from it was immediately trapped by the icy cold from the window. It formed feathery curls of frost on the inside of the glass. The three windowless walls were liberally adorned with evidence of Goatstroke's prominence: honorary degrees from the most prestigious universities in the world, certificates of merit signed by various heads of state, the cover of a magazine bearing the professor's portrait. John remembered the first time he had come to the office as a freshman, how his heart had thrummed when he talked to the great man. Since then he had grown fairly confident in Goatstroke's presence—until a few months ago, when he'd started commuting to Asia and his work had slowed down so dramatically. As he waited for Goatstroke to speak, John realized that he was almost as nervous as he had been during that freshman-year meeting, seven years earlier.

"All right," said Goatstroke, raising his eyes and closing the last page of the article. "How are you, John?"

"I'm fine," John managed to croak.

"Good," said Goatstroke. "Do you have a chapter for me?"

John swallowed. It was a painful procedure. "More or less," he said. He managed to grin as he put the few pages he had written on the professor's desk.

Goatstroke let the papers lie there. "More or less?" he repeated dourly.

John saw that this would not be easy. He had used up virtually every acceptable excuse for his failure to complete his dissertation on his original schedule. Before meeting with Goatstroke, he had already decided that this time he would have to resort to the bare-bones truth.

"We—I mean I—have had some . . . uh . . . interruptions," he said. "Personal things."

Goatstroke's lips went into a thin, tight line as his hand reached reflexively for his beard. Looking at him, John realized that the meeting might go even more badly than he had expected.

"Personal things," said Goatstroke flatly. He raised one eyebrow to indicate that this was a question, if not an open challenge. He was calling John's bluff. All teachers do it. John himself had done it, as a teaching fellow. The usual line went something like, "I'll grant you an extension on a due date if your mother dies, but you'd better be able to show me the body."

John inhaled, painfully. "You know Martha—my wife—is pregnant again."

Goatstroke inclined his head slightly.

"Well, we just found out that she's carrying a Down syndrome baby."

John had been focusing on the window behind the professor's head. Now he looked into the professor's face, to see the reaction. There was none. Goatstroke just sat there, his lips in a line, as if John had said nothing at all.

"They used to call it mongoloidism," said John. He hated the word.

Goatstroke's face curled up as though he had just bitten down on a piece of aluminum foil. His fingers pulled nervously at his beard for a few seconds before he managed to say, "Oh! Terrible!"

John nodded. He could feel tears burning at the backs of his eyes, but he was far from shedding them. It was a tremendous relief to have told someone, face-to-face. John almost began to relax. Fortunately, he had been around Harvard long enough to avoid dropping his guard altogether.

"We just found out yesterday," he said. "I had trouble getting any work done."

Goatstroke nodded. His expression was almost earnest, as open and genuine as John had ever seen it.

"So," said the professor, "I imagine you'll have it taken care of as soon as possible?"

John blinked in confusion. "What do you mean?"

"It is still early enough to take care of the problem," Goatstroke said. "Isn't it?"

"Oh, you mean abortion," said John.

Goatstroke relaxed slightly in his chair.

"No," said John, "we're not going to do that."

At this, Goatstroke's white-tufted jaw dropped slightly. He was generally an inscrutable man; John had never seen him show so much emotion in a single conversation. His face registered both disbelief and outrage.

"Martha wants to have the baby," John finished in a weak voice.

Goatstroke still looked dumbfounded. "For God's sake," he said, "can't you convince her to see reason?"

John blinked some more. His brain seemed to be functioning very slowly. Reason, he thought. See reason. He thought about the voice he had heard in the restaurant. At some level, he'd been thinking about it ever since he had learned about Adam's diagnosis. John himself was not thinking reasonably. He didn't think he had much chance of bringing me around.

"It's not really my decision," he told Goatstroke.

"Yes, but—" Goatstroke had to stop, to collect himself. "Listen," he said. "You have got to persuade her. If not for her career, then for yours."

"Mine?"

"Absolutely." Goatstroke nodded. "John, I'm telling you this not only as your adviser but as someone who hopes one day to call you my colleague. You must convince your wife to do the right thing. Frankly, you've made a lot of choices I consider unwise—but this one is a disaster. If she has that baby, neither one of you will ever get your degrees."

Goatstroke's tone and the look on his face, the way he lowered his head and stared from under his brows straight into John's eyes, made it clear that this was not merely a prediction. It was a threat. John felt as though his stomach had suddenly been removed and his heart had fallen into the empty cavity.

"I don't think . . . ," he began. "I mean, I don't know . . . I don't . . ."

"That's right," said Goatstroke. "You don't." Suddenly, his expression changed. His face took on a look of solemn benevolence. He steepled his fingers together on his desk and leaned forward, pressing his beard to his hands in a gesture that was almost intimate.

"Mr. Beck," he said, lapsing into the formal address he used on undergraduates and other lesser beings, "let me tell you something about myself. When I was an assistant professor, working on my first book and trying to get tenure, my wife—my first wife, that is—discovered she was pregnant."

"Oh," said John.

"I was quite moved, at the time—I mean, it really is quite something, to think that a child with your genes has been conceived. But you see, the timing was all wrong. If that baby had been born, it would have interfered with my writing, my research. I decided that she needed an abortion, and I've never regretted it."

"You decided," John croaked.

"What?" said Goatstroke.

"Nothing."

John was having one of those epiphanies men sometimes get, where for a brief moment they can see what the world must look like through a woman's eyes. He was thinking about the way I pored over my pregnancy books and felt for the baby's hands against my sides and cried at the picture on the ultrasound screen. He wondered how many other decisions Goatstroke had made for his wives.

"You have got to understand," Goatstroke went on, "that this is not some game we're playing. This is your *career*, John. You must have your priorities in order."

He was looking very earnestly at John, but John was having a hard time looking back at him. He could barely focus his eyes. It suddenly seemed to him that he was looking at his mentor from some other place, high up and far away. From this new perspective, Goatstroke's office didn't look nearly so glamorous. The great scholar himself appeared to be nothing more than a small man in a small life. John blinked hard, wondering if he was becoming delirious.

"This is the kind of thing that separates the men from the boys," Goatstroke went on. "When you run up against one of life's obstacles— and we all do, at one time or another—that's when you have to prove yourself. Are you going to make the right choice for your career, or are you going to crumble?"

John gave a docile nod. It suddenly occurred to him that Goatstroke's beard was about the same size and color as a hamster he had once owned. In fact, as he thought about it, Goatstroke reminded John of a hamster. He looked at the stacks of journal articles on the professor's desk. He knew that his mentor's life consisted largely of reading such articles, in order to write other articles almost exactly like them. These would be read only by other academics, who in turn would use them to churn out more. It reminded John of the way a caged hamster could run on its little treadmill, exerting tremendous amounts of energy, staying in exactly the same place. He'd read that a hamster could run up to eight miles a day this way, never moving forward a single inch.

"At least," Goatstroke was saying, "at least you will institutionalize the child once it is born? Surely your religious strictures will allow you that?"

John frowned. "Religious strictures?"

"We might as well be open about it, John. I know your religion forbids abortion."

John was still frowning. "I guess so," he said slowly. "I hadn't thought about it."

Goatstroke shook his head. "The Dark Ages still cast their shadow on the brightest minds."

John thought about trying to convince Goatstroke that my decision to keep Adam had virtually nothing to do with organized religion. In the end, he decided it wasn't worth the pain it would cause his sore throat. The professor didn't seem to have any desire to listen to John's explanation about anything. He was still talking, so John just sat quietly, folding his hands in his lap like a little boy hearing a story.

"I'll be blunt," said Goatstroke. "You've got to get back on track with this dissertation. That should be your complete focus—not worrying about some defective child that doesn't even have to be born."

John nodded again, almost absentmindedly. A peculiar thought had just occurred to him. At first it was just a whisper, like the buzzing of a mosquito. He brushed it away a few times, but it came back, until suddenly it popped into clear focus.

Professor Goatstroke was going to die.

This simple truth struck John with the force of a subway train. He had never thought about Goatstroke's death, not even when it would have saved him from handing in a chapter of his dissertation. It wasn't that the death was imminent, or even in the middle future. The point was not that it was soon, only that it was coming. Inexorably. Inevitably.

John looked around the office again, at the many degrees and honors hanging on the walls. He wondered what comfort the office brought to Goatstroke, whether it helped him through the nights. Maybe the ordinary nights, John decided. The nights when tragedy was comfortably far away, when bad news could be flicked out of the room with the touch of the remote control. But what about the other nights, John wondered, the nights when Goatstroke was ill, when he had lost a friend, when he saw in the mirror that his body was acquiring the stoop-shouldered fragility of an old man? John's head ached mightily as he realized that he, himself, could not have been comforted by anything in that office. Maybe it worked for Goatstroke but not for John. He saw nothing on the professor's walls worth trading for a piece of his life.

Goatstroke had been talking for some time. He paused, frustrated, when he realized that John had barely heard him.

At the sudden silence, John's attention snapped back to the conversation. He cleared his swollen throat. He knew that what he was about to say would ruin him in Goatstroke's eyes. He didn't understand why he was going to say it, why saying it seemed extremely important.

"It's not only Martha," John said. "I mean, it is her choice to make, but I agree with her. I want the baby too."

Goatstroke's reaction, predictable as it was, still stung. John watched the disbelief in the older man's eyes turn to anger, anger at John's decision, and even more, at what amounted to insubordination. It was the first time in their relationship that John had discounted his mentor's advice.

"Well," said Goatstroke curtly. "It's your life. I suppose you can do what you want with it."

"Yes," said John. His head felt numb. He took a final glance around the cramped, dingy office, marveling that he had never put into words how much it looked and felt like a cage.

"I'll read over this," said Goatstroke, picking up the papers John had left on his desk. "I certainly hope it's good enough."

John nodded. He knew it wouldn't be good enough.

They made their formal good-byes, and John turned and left the office, the professor's eyes burning into his back. He stopped for a moment in the hall as the door slowly closed. Through the frosted glass he could see Goatstroke bending toward another article, stroking the little hamster on his chin. Eight miles a day, John thought again, and never moving an inch.

As he took his first few steps away from the office, John felt crushed, stunned by the damage he had wreaked on his own career with a few misplaced words. He began to berate himself for speaking up to Goatstroke—but surprisingly, when he reconsidered the encounter, he didn't feel sorry at all. Instead he had a sensation of the immense weight slowly beginning to slide off him. The farther he got from Goatstroke's office, the lighter he felt. By the time he reached the outside door of the building, he was almost running, his toes bouncing him into the air with very step. He left the building with his head pounding, the soreness in his throat spreading to his lungs, his heart broken, and the wreckage of his fledgling career falling down around his ears. He should have been devastated, he thought. Any sane person would be. But instead, as John emerged into the frozen afternoon and began to sprint along the pathway that led away from Professor Goatstroke's office, he felt more and more as though he were flying.

24

∽ Four days after hearing the diagnosis, I still wasn't able to eat or sleep. My body seemed to have decided not to go forward with any normal functioning until it heard better news. Better news was not to be had. I looked. I looked everywhere. Information about Down syndrome was surprisingly hard to find at Harvard, but I read what I could find with desperate intensity. Later, when the people around me had time to marshal better resources, I would learn a few not-so-awful things about my son's condition. But those first few days, I swallowed thousands of appalling bits of information from insensitive and outdated sources. I swallowed them without even chewing.

I have seen the same sort of craving for information in people who have lost loved ones to illness or injury. They rivet all their attention on the postmortem analysis or the police report or the black box, clinging to the facts of the case as though understanding the cause of death will soften its horrible finality. As far as I can tell, this never really works. When all the data are in, when the case is closed and sealed, the dead are still dead.

My situation in the months before Adam's birth was in some ways better than this, and in other ways worse. On the one hand, I was still having a baby. He still bounced around on my bladder and invited me down for the occasional game of Prod. On the other hand, the more I learned about all the possible problems connected with Down syndrome, the more I became afraid of him. I went into a state of alternating protectiveness and terror toward the baby. Half the time the exploratory thumps from my insides seemed to come from a monster, like that disgusting creature in the movie *Alien* that rips its way out of a crew member's abdomen and sets out to eat every human it encounters. Then, just when I was ready to lose my mind, I would accidentally glance at the ultrasound picture of Adam floating around in the amniotic fluid like a

212 _ Martha Beck

perfect, sweet-faced doll, and feel a love so strong it shattered the fear like a pure, high tone shatters crystal. Then I would set out to read more about Down syndrome, by way of becoming a better mother, and the fear would begin to harden all over again.

The little mustard-yellow book I'd bought at the Coop was the worst. It had last been updated in about 1950, when people with Down syndrome were rarely seen outside of institutions. I understand now, and I want to state for the record, that putting a person with Down's into an institution is like forcing an otter to live in a Pringle's can. There is nothing wrong with the social adaptability of people like Adam. They are as gregarious as any "normal" person, more so than many, and thrive on loving interaction. They also learn social skills as quickly as any child, given normal treatment. It makes me sick to think of the thousands of children who were raised in institutions before the last couple of decades. Isolated, bored, and aching with loneliness, many literally turned their faces to the wall and died by the time they were in their teens or early twenties. The mustard book described this as the normal life course for the human beings it called "mongoloid idiots."

Oh, that book was full of tasty treats for the parent of a child with Down's. I've met hundreds of parents whose decisions about their children's lives were made on the basis of such incredible misinformation. My book declared grandly that the birth of a Down syndrome child generally destroyed the mother's mental health, as well as the life of any older sisters that might be in the family (brothers, it said, were exempt, since they were not expected to fill a caretaking role). It gave absolutely false information about the inability of such children to control their bodily functions, and their antisocial inclinations. It listed the typical IQ for "mongoloids" as about 35, and by way of comparison, mentioned that the IQ of a chimpanzee is about 50 and that of the average *oak tree* is 3. (I don't know how you'd test the IQ of an oak tree, but apparently the authors of this particular book got one to answer at least a few questions.) It was impossible for me to keep myself from calculating that this meant my son's IQ would be about 130 points below the average of my oft tested siblings, and only 32 points higher than the plants in Harvard Yard.

A year later, when we had moved to Utah and I was doing research for my dissertation, I ran across that mustard-yellow book in a box of reference materials. By that time, Adam was an adventurous, affectionate little boy who loved to draw, tickle his sister, and explore all our floor-level kitchen cabinets. I had learned a great deal about the fear and mis-judgment that had been leveled at people with Down syndrome for so many years. Just a glance at that book yanked me abruptly back to the days after Adam's diagnosis, when I hadn't learned any of these things, when I'd forced myself to read and accept claims that were both untrue and brutally unkind. Before I was aware of having moved, I slammed that book across the room so hard that pages flew like feathers when it hit the wall. I chased it down, grabbed it, and tore it straight across and then down the middle, with the same kind of fevered strength that enables a mother to lift a life-crushing weight, like a tractor or a stereotype, off her pinned and struggling child.

In the days following Adam's diagnosis, however, I seemed to have no strength at all. I made a halfhearted effort at sleeping but barely even tried to eat. It had been difficult enough before, with the nausea killing my appetite. Once I heard about the Down syndrome, it simply became impossible. After four days of numbness and physical decline, I finally admitted to myself that I probably needed another IV. It wasn't as if this was a new idea—I'd been getting them regularly for months—but the thought of going back to University Health Services was almost unbear-able. The place had become so aversive to me that I would go blocks out of my way to avoid walking past it. It took a lot of misery to get me to the point of going inside and mentioning that I was, once again, dehy-drated. I felt like a plant that had to be watered every few days. An oak tree, perhaps.

Nevertheless, it was with considerable relief that I finally lay down on one of the clinic's two beds and allowed yet another fledgling Florence Nightingale to try to lace the IV needle into my legendary veins. They were so limp from dehydration that this particular nurse punctured all the available forearm locations and ended up inserting the drip in my ankle. I didn't mind at all, though, because before she even got started with the needle, she read my chart and turned to me with a look of such compassion that it almost unhinged me. Then she set her cool, soft hand on mine and whispered, "He's going to be a beautiful baby. I have a brother." This is the way families who have an Adam talk to each other, in a gentle, indirect language that requires very little explanation. I cried the whole time that nurse was there, and it had nothing to do with needles.

By the time the glucose solution had begun to plump up my veins and my head cleared a little, it was 8:00 P.M. and dark as death outside. The admitting physician had recommended that I spend the night at the infirmary, to see if I would be able to hold down food once my stores of electrolytes were replenished, so I settled in and prepared to try to sleep.

The infirmary was a small room with four beds, steel ones, bolted to warped linoleum under harsh fluorescent lights. I had been there twice before, once when a friend of mine sicked out of a test by eating a bar of soap, and again when one of John's roommates had developed some sort of psychogenic paralysis, also because of exam anxiety. That infirmary filled right up around exam time. The night I stayed there, however, was near the beginning of the spring semester, and the room was nearly empty. There was only one patient besides me, a woman named Maude, who worked in the dormitory kitchens. Maude had an extraordinarily thick Boston accent and a face like a lump of bread dough, from which her eyes peered like inset raisins. She told me that she was in the infirmary because she was unable to pee without a catheter. The doctors were trying to figure out why.

Maude voiced my own feeling that the fluorescent lighting was extremely unpleasant. After pressing our "call nurse" buttons for a while with no result, we decided that I should get out of bed and hop over to switch it off, holding my plugged-in ankle carefully so as not to rip out the IV. My mission accomplished, Maude switched on a little reading light she had brought from home, casting a small yellow glow. "Is this going to keep you awake, Mather deah?" she asked kindly.

I shook my head and closed my eyes. My body was feeling better as it absorbed liquid, but my soul hurt so much I could hardly talk. I didn't think I would be able to sleep.

"I'm just going to stay awake," said Maude, "because I have a visitor coming. I'm helping my friend study for the bar exam."

I opened one eye and said, "Oh. That's good."

I was a little surprised that Maude should be helping someone become an attorney, then immediately berated myself for being so classist. Still, I was surprised again when Maude's friend showed up. I had expected another woman, maybe someone Maude's age who had decided to go back to school. The friend turned out to be a huge, twenty-something African-American man named Emory, who wore so much jewelry that it jingled faintly whenever he moved. Maude didn't introduce us; she thought I was asleep, which was fine with me. I watched through my eyelashes as Emory pulled the visitor's chair close to Maude's bed and handed her a book.

"Okay," he said. "Quiz me."

At the sound of his voice, I opened my eyes all the way and looked at him in wonder. It was one of those almost inhumanly beautiful voices, like the deep, echoing hum of a cello played softly. Emory kept his voice down, to avoid waking me, and I found that just by concentrating on his lovely voice, I could go to that soothing, half-conscious state between waking and sleeping. To this day, whenever I get a little anxious, I go back to the sound of Emory's voice.

"Wheah should I staht, deah?" said Maude.

"Anywhere," Emory told her.

"All right, then," she said. "Margarita."

There was a pause before Emory said, "Three parts tequila, one part triple sec, juice from half a lime. Salt the glass rim. Frozen or on the rocks."

They weren't looking at me, over in my darkened corner of the room. This was good, because I'm not sure exactly what expression showed up on my face as I realized that when Maude had said "bar exam," she'd meant *bar* exam.

"Whiskey sour," she said, and Emory responded, "Four parts rye whiskey, one part lemon juice, a teaspoon of sugar. Garnish with a maraschino cherry and a slice of orange."

That was the first time since Adam's diagnosis that I had been yanked out of my introverted despair and into a kind of lightheartedness. I remembered my older sister, in the midst of a hellish divorce, mentioning that life would be completely unbearable if it weren't so hilarious. I began to laugh under my breath, and then the tears came again, and I began to relax. The sound of Emory's voice, listing the mellifluous recipes for various alcoholic drinks, soothed me to sleep like a lullaby.

The next morning I was awakened by four doctors, who marched into the room in a vaguely military procession. Three of them looked young and were unfamiliar to me; the fourth was one of the many doctors connected to the clinic's obstetrical unit. This doctor, whom I will call Grendel, was a popular topic of conversation among the women who came to University Health Services for their prenatal care. Everyone wanted Grendel to be on call when they actually delivered their babies. He was supposed to be a wonder in the delivery room: gracious and concerned and incredibly skillful. However, no one wanted to have Grendel conduct her prenatal exams. He apparently didn't think much of these routine appointments, and his bedside manner tended to be aloof, if not downright disdainful.

I myself had been examined by Grendel only once, about three months into my pregnancy. I was used to chatting a little with the doctors before the actual exam, on the old-fashioned grounds that it's nice to be on speaking terms with a person before you allow him or her unlimited access to your genital region. When I'd spoken to Grendel, he'd look at me with an expression of disgust and answered not a word. During the entire exam, he remained silent except to ask me medical questions. He never looked at my face or smiled. He left me with the impression that I was distinctly unworthy of his time and attention. Judging from what other patients said about their appointments with Grendel, this seemed to have been his usual demeanor.

I was therefore very surprised to see Grendel approach my bed in the infirmary that morning, trailing his three disciples. The younger physicians lined up against the wall beside my bed, while Grendel walked right up and peered earnestly into my eyes. He was short, with very thick glasses, through which his eyes peered with peculiar intensity, and the skin on his face was very tight, as though it had been stretched across his bones. He had no visible lips.

I blinked, pulling myself awake, wondering what Dr. Grendel was doing at my bedside. At some level, I jumped to the conclusion that since mine was now officially a "high-risk" pregnancy, Dr. Grendel had decided it was worth his time. I felt a surge of relief, knowing his reputation as a superb obstetrician and believing that, somehow, his presence would give my baby a better chance.

"Good morning, Martha," said Grendel. I was amazed. He virtually never addressed his patients at all, much less by their first names. His voice was friendly and kind, with a little sadness around the edges.

"Morning," I said.

"Do you mind if I sit down?" The only visitor's chair was still over by Maude. Grendel patted the foot of my bed, and I nodded. He sat down sidesaddle.

"How are you feeling?" he asked.

I thought about it. "Better," I said. "I'm not sure I'll be able to keep down any food, but I feel like I could try."

Grendel nodded, the skin on his neck relaxing and then stretching tight again. "Your chart says that you haven't eaten for four days."

I felt myself blush, embarrassed. "I know. I tried."

Grendel gave a long sigh, looking away from me and down at the toes of his shoes.

"We all know what you're trying to do," he said gently.

I glanced at the three young doctors, who were looking on with apparent interest. "You do?" I said. I myself didn't know what I was trying to do. I was hoping they could tell me.

"There are more efficient ways to take care of this problem than starving yourself until the fetus dies," said Grendel.

I stared at him. "Excuse me?"

"Martha, it's obvious," he said. He looked at me again, his face suddenly stern. "Why else would you stop eating?"

For a minute I just opened and closed my mouth without making any noise, like a fish. Then I said, "But I've been sick all along. And I'm upset, and—"

"Exactly," Grendel cut in. "You're upset. I think it's time to let us take care of it for you."

I was getting the picture. I felt myself go cold inside, as though I had swallowed liquid nitrogen.

"Martha, listen to me," said Grendel urgently. His piercing little eyes were full of concern. "I have been in this business for a very long time. I've had several cases like yours, and in every case, the woman has made . . . uh . . . the other decision."

I was beginning to tremble. I wished that I had my clothes on, instead of the hospital napkin. I didn't know what to say.

"You are also the youngest woman I have ever dealt with on this particular problem," said Grendel. He paused meaningfully, glancing up at the three student doctors arrayed along the wall.

It took me a second to catch on. Then I said, "You think I'm making this decision because I'm too young to know better?"

Grendel didn't even look at me. He and the three disciples nodded at each other.

I felt dizzy, overwhelmed. It was true that I was young and inexperienced, but the chief effect that I could see was that I didn't know how to assert myself with world-renowned obstetricians.

"You realize," Grendel went on, "that you are placing a very heavy burden on yourself and your entire family. Did you know that eighty percent of couples who have a child with this condition end up divorcing?"

I swallowed, though my mouth was very dry. "No," I said. "I didn't know that."

"I would not make the choice that you have made," he went on steadily. "I have never known anyone who would."

The other doctors were watching me intently, as if I were a tree that Grendel was chopping down and they were waiting to see me topple.

"I don't know," I mumbled. "I guess I just . . . I just can't reject him."

It was a miserably inadequate statement. My real feeling, the one I couldn't articulate yet, was that my entire life hinged on knowing that there were people who would continue to love me unconditionally, even if I were damaged, even if I were sick. Such love was the only thing that had sustained me during the turmoil of the past months. If I eliminated my child because of his disability, if I put him out of my life, I would be violating the only thing that was keeping me alive. I'd be ripping the rug out from under my own feet.

Grendel was looking at me with obvious frustration. The skin across his cheekbones tightened even more as he pursed his lips.

"Well, I can't do the operation against your will," he said. "Of course, if a patient came in here with a malignant tumor and refused to let me remove it, I couldn't do that operation either. Even if we all knew what was best."

The other doctors nodded.

It is difficult to convey the fear and despair I felt as the weight of their collective disapproval bore down on me. It was like a wall of ice backing me slowly into a corner. I could hardly breathe. I remember wishing desperately that Dr. Grendel would move away from me, get off the bed, give me some space.

Since that time, beginning a few months after Adam's birth, I have addressed a number of medical conferences on the topic of ethics related to the new obstetrical technologies. My firm opinion is that women should be given all relevant medical information and then allowed to make up their own minds about whether or not to abort their fetuses. Invariably, I am approached after these conferences by doctors—never nurses, always doctors—who disagree with me. They argue quite explicitly that they are highly trained professionals, that their opinions are far more informed than the average pregnant woman's, and that they are therefore in a much better position to make the right decision about any particular woman's abortion than the woman herself. Some of these physicians are pro-lifers who would never abort a fetus with Down syndrome, others would do so without exception. I would like to take this opportunity to invite all such doctors (and I recognize that they represent a minority of their profession) to fold it five ways and put it where the sun don't shine.

Oh, I'm sorry—do I sound a little bitter? Hm. Perhaps that's because, in the years since that encounter with Dr. Grendel, I have had so many physicians wedge their personal prejudices into my life, into Adam's life, and call it medical advice. Dr. Grendel, who had never seen a woman elect to keep a Down syndrome baby, was as ignorant as the most severely retarded child when it came to the actual consequences of my choice. I doubt very much that he had ever really known anyone with Down syndrome. I'd bet my life he'd never loved such a person.

I once spoke to an entering class of Harvard Medical School students about my pregnancy and my decision. Adam was asleep on my lap at the time, wearing a bow tie and a dreamy expression. After the speech, I was approached by an elderly professor whose name I forget. He had just become the grandfather of a little girl with Down's. As he talked to me, he stroked Adam's soft blond hair and wept. He loved his granddaughter with inexplicable openness, and the experience had changed his whole life. Now there's a doctor with some real information to offer the parents of a retarded baby. Whoever said that love is blind was dead wrong. Love is the only thing on this earth that lets us see each other with the remotest accuracy.

I suppose that I am grateful to Dr. Grendel for showing me so explicitly the prejudice of the Harvard medical community. I called the nurse-practitioner after he left, to ask if any of the other obstetricians connected with Harvard were in favor of my decision to continue the pregnancy. She didn't think so. So after that morning visit, I knew where I stood. Most, if not all, of the doctors I would interact with for the remainder of my pregnancy disagreed with my decision; would have considered it wiser to do away with the baby they were helping me protect. An awkward situation, to be sure.

At the time that Dr. Grendel sat on my bed and tried to talk some sense into me, it was almost more than I could bear. After all, I was a good girl, a conscientious student, a high achiever. I always did what the grown-ups said to do, especially when they were prestigious and successful grown-ups. I knew that I was still certain I didn't want an abortion, but I was completely unskilled in the practice of disagreeing with an authority figure—let alone a whole *team* of authority figures like Grendel and the Go-Gos.

Fortunately, the puppeteers were there.

Grendel was launching into a recitation of various horrible things about children with Down syndrome when that voice—the calm, inaudible voice I had heard a few times before—drowned out the doctor's voice with a simple question.

Why is he doing this?

I looked at Grendel closely, suddenly feeling like an observer rather than a patient. Why, indeed. This man always made a great show of being too busy even to look at his patients. Why was he spending this inordinate amount of time trying to convince me to abort a child he would probably never even see?

As I considered this question, a strange thing began to happen. It was a little bit like the Seeing Thing, in that I had a visual impression of something that wasn't physically there. But I wasn't seeing across distance this time. I was seeing through facades. I looked at Grendel's face, and there, just behind the tight-stretched skin, I seemed to see another face appear. It was Grendel, but not the wise and solemn physician who was displaying his technique to the three students. This face was terrified. The fear in its eyes were heavily laced with pain, old pain, pain so deep it had become a way of life.

Grendel was scared to death.

This kind of seeing has happened to me many times since. I believe it happens to everyone. It happens when you meet some smiling person and walk away with the distinct impression that the person means you no good. It happens when a teenager lashes out at you, and instead of anger you suddenly see the bewildered battle he is fighting inside himself. It happens when you strike up an acquaintance and, within fifteen minutes, know you have made a friend. I believe our intuition is far more delicate, and accurate, than we allow ourselves to admit. I had to be pushed to the brink of complete breakdown before I let myself trust mine, or even notice what it was telling me. But that day in the infirmary, it was so incredibly vivid, so visual, that it stunned me. My fear of Grendel was completely gone. The doctor was like a bee, a snake, a dog; he was attacking me only because he felt that I threatened his survival.

Why should this be? I relaxed and looked frankly at the second face that drifted, panicky and bewildered, behind Grendel's strange, taut skin. I examined this new face with some care. The fear in it spoke to me of a lifetime spent desperately avoiding the stigma of stupidity, of failure, of not measuring up. I knew plenty of premeds at Harvard, and as a group, I think they were even more obsessed than the rest of us with climbing to the very top of the prestige heap. They were famous for things like razoring out the pages in the reserved readings for their courses, so that none of their classmates could study the material. It was said that it took two Harvard premeds to change a lightbulb, one to change the bulb and the other to push the ladder out from under him. Dr. Grendel had fought his way through the increasingly rarefied ranks of such people to achieve the apex of his profession. Something had driven him all that way, and it wasn't just affection for his patients. I was convinced, looking at his fear-face, that Grendel's entire philosophy of life centered on obliterating the stupid little boy inside him. It was that person he feared, desperately feared, and this was why he was begging so earnestly for a chance to obliterate the stupid little boy inside me.

I looked at Grendel, and I looked at his acolytes. They, too, had their fears and their agendas. It was obvious to me as I looked through the new set of eyes Adam had given me. As Grendel finished his closing arguments, I stretched out to my full length on the bed, pushing the doctor slightly aside with my feet.

"Thank you," I said. "You can go now."

Grendel and the gang stared at me in frustration and disbelief. The doctor chewed his lip with obvious anxiety, the fear-face trembling under his physical visage like that of a man facing execution. Eventually, he heaved a huge sigh and rubbed his hands together emphatically, making a clear point to the other doctors that he was washing his hands of this matter, once and for all. As they filed out of the room, Adam gave me a cheerful wallop just below the navel. Grendel was last in line, and before he left, his fear-face, though not his flesh-and-blood head, turned to look behind him with those terrified eyes. I could see the fear, as clear as day, but I didn't feel it. Briefly, for the first time since I had bought the mustard-yellow book and started soaking in the prejudices against the developmentally disabled world, I was not afraid at all.

25

⮂   When Adam was a little bitty critter, about two years old and not yet twenty pounds, our whole family went for a ride on the World's Steepest Skytram. The Skytram was located near our home in the Rocky Mountains. John had just received his Ph.D. and was teaching at the university where both our fathers worked, while I wrote my dissertation. There weren't many exciting things to do in that region of the country, but the Skytram was definitely one of them. It was basically a Plexiglas box hanging from a cable, with seats for passengers inside. It went up from a canyon streambed to the top of a minor mountain peak, rising about a thousand feet in less than half a mile. It looked pretty darn near vertical even from ground level, and when you actually got in the box and it started chugging its way up, any fear of heights you may ever have possessed tapped you politely on the shoulder and said, "What the hell do you think you're doing?"

The most frightening thing about the Skytram experience was that the floor of the box was as clear as glass. Looking out the side windows was slightly unnerving in itself, but the first time you glanced down and saw all that nothingness gaping below you was truly a religious experience. I myself am no more bothered by heights than the average person. I'm not afraid to fly, and I've rappelled down sheer cliff faces without hesitation or alarm. But that day on the Skytram—when I first saw my *children* sitting on slick plastic seats above a sheer drop to the whitewater rapids below us—there was a moment when I seriously questioned whether Adam was the only one in the family who needed a diaper.

Adam was sitting on John's lap. He was going through a phase of farsightedness, which is common in kids with Down's, and he was wearing these little glasses that magnified his eyes. They made him appear very solemn and wise, especially for one so diminutive. As we rose from ground level, Adam was captivated by the view of the mountain peaks

224

around us. He pointed and babbled as we passed huge evergreen trees and outcroppings of stone. Then, absentmindedly, he looked down. I happened to be watching him at the time. He froze the second his gaze fell to the invisible floor, and his eyes went huge behind his glasses. For a few long seconds he sat completely still in John's lap, staring downward and taking deep breaths, as if trying to collect himself. Then his expression changed, as though he had come to some sort of conclusion. He reached out one tiny, chubby hand, put it under John's chin, and pushed up as hard as he could.

"Whatcha doing, Adam?" said John, pulling his head back.

Adam had to turn toward John's body and struggle to his knees in order to keep his hand under John's chin. Once he was firmly in position, he reached his other hand over to me and tried to push my chin up, too. At that time, Adam was still years away from his first word. I didn't know whether he had ever experienced anything like an abstract thought, or whether he was just a frisky, farsighted form of vegetable life. In this context it was startling to realize how clearly Adam had evaluated the situation on the Skytram, and how he'd decided to respond to it. He was protecting us. He didn't seem to fear looking down himself, but he wanted to spare John and me the terror of dangling out in space with no visible means of support. Adam clearly knew, even then, that he was much better at handling anxiety than either of his parents.

Looking back on the Skytram experience, I am particularly struck by how solicitous Adam was of John. My husband is not the kind of person who shows his fears easily. As I've already said, he hid his vulnerabilities better than most people I encountered at Harvard—and that's saying something. I know John as well as anyone on earth, and even I often can't see through his nonchalant exterior to any fears that may be lurking inside. But Adam can. He can read John like big red letters on a neon sign. He knew perfectly well, that day on the Skytram, that letting his father stare down at the whitewater so far below us would have been a serious mistake.

The sensation I had on that tram was very like the feeling I lived with during the last few months before Adam was born. I kept moving inexorably toward having the baby, my body growing, my mind disintegrating. As far as I can tell, my connection to reality was about as tenuous as that pathetic little cable stretched between streambed and cliff. Unfortunately, Adam was not yet in a position to keep me from focusing my full attention on every possible danger. I "looked down," so to speak, the whole damn time. I sat around brooding and worrying and grieving as though I'd forgotten how to do anything else, because I had. I didn't sleep well, couldn't eat much, cried frequently. I leaned heavily on the care and generosity of Sibyl and Deirdre and other friends. I grieved less openly around these people than I did when I was alone, but when the chips were down, I knew that it was all right to show how much pain I was feeling.

John, by contrast, was Mr. Stoicism. His mother kindly confided in me about the loss of her own first and fourth babies, neither of whom lived long enough for John to know them. I was comforted to know I was not the only mother who had ever grieved, but I was also amazed at my mother-in-law's pioneer toughness. She never got so much as a quaver in her voice as she described her babies' deaths. This was John's family legacy—and John, we must remember, is a guy. A male of the species. Whatever changes the last few decades have wrought on our culture's expectations of fatherhood, it doesn't take a Beck to know that Real Men don't sit around oozing tears and fears in relation to unborn babies. A Real Man stays out working or drinking while his wife throws the calf; then he waits a few years, takes the kid out to the corral, and teaches him to fight. Without crying. The very thought of crying makes a Real Man want to hawk up a big gob of tobacco juice and spit it on your shoes.

It was especially difficult for John to take in any of the emotional impact of Adam's diagnosis when there was so much to be done just maintaining our family. Much later, John would admit to me that the only way he managed to keep going, to keep getting up after two hours of sleep and working on his dissertation and taking care of Katie and dragging me to the hospital for refills and preparing consulting presentations and holding me while I cried and all the rest of it, was to pretend that nothing was happening except the immediate task before him. For the last third of my pregnancy, John didn't really believe that we had a baby coming, let alone a retarded one. He couldn't. It would have been too much for him. This coping mechanism got him—got us—through that time. It also led to a lot of arguments.

"Look, Martha," John would say when he found me snuffling and dripping on yet another open textbook, "it's really time you got over this and got on with your life."

"Got *over* it?" I would sob. "How can you even *say* that? Doesn't this bother you at *all*?" (I talked in italics a lot during that time.)

John would look at me thoughtfully for a minute, and then he would say, "No, not really," with the serene conviction of a man in complete denial.

"It *doesn't*?" I'd gasp. "Why not? Why in God's name *not*? How can you *be* this way?"

"I just think about something else," John would explain patiently. "You should, too. Then maybe you wouldn't get so hysterical."

"Just think about something *else*?" I'd shout, almost frothing at the mouth. "Okay, tough guy, let's try this—I'll get a retarded person to kick *you* in the stomach every thirty seconds, and then we'll see how easy it is for *you* to *think about something else*!"

In short, as Grendel the obstetrician had promised me, the whole Adam thing was getting very hard on our marriage. It was years before I realized how close I came to losing John just when I needed him most. Since he was a Real Man, or at least doing a reasonably good impression of a Real Man, I actually believed that all the chaos I felt in my own life wasn't really bothering him. Adam was about four or five before John told me that when he left for Asia in March of 1988, he had pretty much decided he wasn't coming back.

It was a long trip: ten days in Singapore, another three in Japan. During the Singapore phase, while he was working with the other consultants, John felt like a wounded old man at a high school pep rally. His heart felt too tired to beat, his lungs to breathe. Instead of racing ahead of everyone else at work, as he was accustomed to doing, he had to force himself to keep pace. During lunch breaks, when his colleagues headed off to a restaurant or bar, he would excuse himself and set out for endless, aimless walks through the muggy streets of Singapore. He came home with a brick-red upper body where the tropical sun had burnt him through the fabric of his shirt, except for a pale arrow in the shape of his tie down the center of his chest. It must have been incredibly uncomfortable to wander so long in that suffocating climate, but John didn't notice it. He was so far gone he didn't feel much of anything.

I was in close contact with him during that trip, although we didn't talk much on the phone. The Seeing Thing happened to me intermittently the whole time. It didn't surprise me; in fact, I had come to expect it. One day, when I had slipped into that half-conscious state between sleeping and waking, I dreamed of a great, gray, growling creature, like a Chinese dragon. It had translucent skin, through which its veins showed in vivid white flashes. This strange image cheered me up. I'd done my undergraduate thesis on Chinese folklore, so I knew that the year Adam would be born, the Year of the Dragon, was the most auspicious of birth signs. When a mother dreams of dragons, it sends a very positive message about her baby.

A few hours later, John called from Japan to tell me that he had just flown over the Philippines during a midnight thunderstorm. It was, he said, as strange and beautiful a sight as he had ever seen. The lightning flashing within the smoky clouds had lit them with brilliant, jagged lines, white and blue and faintly pink. I remember feeling a moment of genuine disappointment that the mental image I had seen was not a Chinese omen but merely a telepathic transmission from my husband, ten thousand miles away. It is at times like these that one realizes just how far off the deep end one has really gone.

Whenever the Seeing Thing happened during that trip, the emotion that came with it was one of almost unendurable sadness. I believed— still do—that the sadness I felt during those moments was actually John's. What I didn't know was that he was not simply grieving the loss of our son's normalcy, as I was doing. He was on the verge of something even more drastic. John had not yet articulated it to himself, but in a wordless, deadened way, he knew that he was about to make a choice.

He knew that he *should* return to Cambridge and pick up his many burdens, as he had been trained to do, without question or complaint. But what he *wanted* to do was stay in Asia, perhaps move into a full-time position with his company's Asian office. If worse came to worst and the firm didn't need him there, he could always teach English in Japan until he got a better job. He would send money back to me and Katie and the Monster Fetus, and then later—much later, when the baby was a known quantity and John was well rested again—we could all join him overseas.

From John's perspective, there were many things to recommend this plan. Long-distance relationships, with separations of years' duration, are not uncommon among international executives and their spouses. John knew that he could make enough money as a full-time consultant to support me and the children comfortably, even though he wouldn't be physically near us. And then there was the conviction that Professor Goatstroke had firmly implanted in John's mind: that if Adam actually made it to being born (but not as far as entering an institution), John would never earn his degree. All his years of work and sacrifice, all his hopes for his future career, would come to nothing. It was an overwhelming thought. When he was tired and stressed, which was always, it heavily outweighed the memory of the strange voice that had told him, *John, keep the baby.* Listening to the voice was manifestly ridiculous. In the final analysis, staying in Asia, doing on-site research, and freeing himself from all but financial responsibility for his family seemed to John the only possible way to prove his commitment to his work and become truly Successful.

The worst part of the plan was the thought of leaving me alone with two very dependent children. But deep in his gut, John had reached the anger stage of the grieving process, and much of his anger was directed at me. In a very real way, I was the one who had chosen to make our lives so hard. I had unilaterally decided to keep the baby, early on when I realized I was pregnant and later, when we knew about the Down syndrome. John was not one to butt in on a woman's right to make her own choices in such matters. Nevertheless, he felt profoundly helpless and disempowered. There were two or three times after the amniocentesis results came back that John hinted around about how awful it was to have so little say in something that affected him so profoundly. I responded by narrowing my eyes and asking him if he liked feeling the way women have felt throughout history, at almost all times and all places. This tended to close down the discussion pretty quickly, leaving John's feelings unaired and his preferences rebuffed without any hearing at all, let alone a fair one.

So it was that on a chilly evening in March, John sat in a Tokyo jazz bar and toyed with the idea of boarding a plane for Singapore, instead of Los Angeles, the next morning. He had gone to the bar to hear the blues, which were being sung with skill and passion by a little Japanese man in a fez. It was a deeply incongruous scene. Nevertheless, it helped John get through his numbness. He sat in the dark, amid packed-in Japanese customers, and began to feel things for the first time in weeks. Then he immediately and devoutly wished he could go numb again. His feelings, from the ache in his head to the guilt and sorrow in his heart, were all but unbearable. John dropped his head into his hands and sat there aching. The people around him politely pretended not to notice. The Japanese are good at that.

John was not drunk when he left the bar, but he might as well have been. The melting pot of pan-Pacific germs in his body, combined with fatigue and topped off by a hefty dose of despair, made him stagger back and forth on the narrow sidewalk like a long-term alcoholic. It was past midnight and very cool. The light of a bright half-moon shone on the narrow, labyrinthine streets. John set out along those streets, not caring where he went, just putting his legs in motion. The motion, the sense of physically running away, came as a great relief.

He still hadn't made up his mind what he should do about his future. No matter how many times he went over it, staying in Asia seemed like the only rational option. Rationality, of course, was the essence of a Harvard man, but the rational course ahead of him wrenched his emotions so hard he thought it might destroy him. On the other hand, the thought of going back to the wreckage of his life in Cambridge was intolerable. John stopped thinking and sped up a little. He had no idea where he was going; he just wanted to move away from where he was. It seemed advisable to continue walking until he either felt better or fell over dead.

John wandered for hours, away from the posh thoroughfares near the jazz bar, past the light and noise of other popular nightspots, through centuries-old streets so narrow he could touch buildings on both sides simultaneously with the tips of his outstretched fingers. The previous summer, when we'd lived in Tokyo, I had managed to get spectacularly lost almost every time I walked out of the house. John never did. This was due partly to an excellent innate sense of direction and partly to the fact that he had spent some of his Mormon mission in Tokyo. John remembered his mission as he trudged through the city eight years later. The thought made him wince. He had known so pathetically little then, had been nothing more than a teenager with decent linguistic ability and an unquestioning obedience to the norms of his parents and his community. He'd fallen in love with Japan, but he hadn't really been able to study its culture and history until he'd returned to Harvard as an Asian studies major.

As he walked, John wondered dully what the streets of Tokyo had sounded like when thousands of wooden sandals had clopped along them, what the city had looked like when the great Japanese heroes had lived. Their names rolled through his mind as he walked: Fukuzawa, Shibusawa, Iwasaki. It suddenly occurred to John that during their lifetimes, none of these men had been sure of his place in history—no more sure than the competitors and enemies they had beaten in their rise to power. It had never occurred to John that these people might have felt vulnerable to failure. And he had never quite realized that the losers of those historic times, the men who had faded into failure and oblivion, had probably started out expecting to win.

It might have been two o'clock in the morning when John finally got too tired to stand up, or it might have been four. He had long ago stopped keeping track of the time—or of his route, although he had a vague idea which of Tokyo's many discrete regions he had reached. He was standing by a row of tiny, close-set houses. On the other side of the narrow street, a high stone wall presented a featureless front. John made his way along the wall until he came to a sort of doorway. As he had expected, the opening in the wall was occupied by an H-shaped gateway. It was the design that leads into most Shinto shrines.

John limped inside the wall. His right knee hurt, and he had a large blister on the opposite heel from walking so far in dress shoes. He was shivering, either from the coolness of the spring air or from fever. John didn't really care. He knew he wanted to sit down, and he didn't really feel capable of thinking beyond that.

The shrine held a simple rock garden bordered with cherry trees, lovingly tended. The cherry trees—*sakura*—were already beginning to bloom. John could have smelled them if his nose and sinuses hadn't been clogged for what seemed like most of his life. In the center of the courtyard was a small temple, really nothing more than a room set on stilts. A gong hung from the roof beam. Someone had placed a long chain of origami paper cranes, symbols of life and hope, near the gong. The rest of the shrine was bedecked with small strips of white paper on which people had written their prayers. John remembered how, as a missionary, he had watched the Japanese stand in front of such temples with their paper strips and clap their hands to get the attention of the gods. He and the other missionaries had often frequented the shrines, hoping to find people desperate enough to believe that a new religion, a strange American one, might be the answer to their problems.

John thought back to the people he had actually converted, to the things he had told them with absolute, nineteen-year-old sincerity. He had told anxious high school students that "the Holy Ghost will bring all things to your remembrance" during their excruciatingly difficult exams. He had parroted memorized scripts about optimism and eternal life to people whose wounded, suspicious eyes had witnessed the wholesale devastation of a lost war. He had promised people maimed and damaged by that war that his God would heal their bodies and their minds. Now, standing in the shrine, John wanted to track down every person he had ever spoken to during his missionary days and tell them he was sorry. He had not understood. He'd been callow, ignorant, insensitive, and wrong.

There was a bench near the pathway that led up to the temple. It was made of stone, upholstered in moss, and rubbed smooth by centuries of use. John walked over to it. On the way, he stopped and faced the temple. He clapped his hands sharply, three times, bowed as tradition dictated, then raised the middle fingers of both hands toward whatever gods happened to be looking on. Then he lay down on the stone surface—on his side, as he had seen homeless beggars do—and closed his eyes.

Later, when John described what happened next, he called it "a dream—sort of." I recognized that ambivalence. I'd had the same uncertainty about the unusual things I'd seen and felt since Adam's conception. They had a dreamlike quality, but at the same time they were vivid enough to seem more real than waking experience. I understand that Jung used to call these "big dreams." John's "big dreams," that night in the shrine, started as nightmares. He dreamt of fires, avalanches, and earthquakes, of horrible accidents he could see coming but had no power to prevent. The emotions he had stored away, ignored, or run from over the past few weeks surged around him like floodwater, drowning him in rage and grief, but especially in fear. The destruction in the nightmares seemed simultaneously random and malignant, absolutely indifferent to the pain it caused but nonetheless carefully planned.

John fought to wake up, to come out of the dream, but could only pull himself to the same place, just below consciousness, where I had seen the storm-dragon. The horrors in his mind's eye continued, but at the same time John began to be aware of his physical surroundings. He also sensed the beginnings of an unfamiliar calm. It was not simply absence of fear but an active calm, a peace of enormous strength. It seemed to emanate from everything around John, from the ancient walls, from the stone and moss beneath his head, from the string of paper cranes swaying in the slight breeze.

John stopped shivering. He felt his body relax completely, a sensation he had all but forgotten. The nightmare was still running, but now he observed it with curious detachment, as though he had taken a few steps back to the cheap seats in his own mind. He felt as if he were watching some sort of game, looking down from the stands. Moreover, he was not alone. There was someone watching with him, a dear friend, someone he had known his entire life—no, more than that. Forever. The companionship John felt with this person was so strong it brought tears to his eyes.

"Look at this," John said in his dream, as the devastation continued to play out before him. "It's horrible. It's too horrible."

The presence beside him smiled. John could feel it. "No, it isn't so horrible," said the being. "It depends on what you want to see. Look."

In the dream, two jumbo jets had just collided in midair, raining twisted metal and fire and broken bodies on the ground below. But when John looked more closely, he could see that every piece of wreckage was transformed as it hit the ground. All the debris was recombining, slowly growing into an airport. The people who had been killed in the collision were walking through the new buildings, boarding the new planes.

"You see," said the presence beside John, "they are going places they could never have reached before. It's not so bad, really. It's just that you don't understand how it works."

Then, suddenly, John's eyes snapped open and he was fully awake. The dream was gone. But the calm was not. Now that he was alert, it had actually gotten stronger. He could feel it almost humming from the rocks and papers and cherry trees. He could smell the scent of the *sakura,* so sweet it was almost intoxicating, and he realized that his nose had cleared. In fact, he felt considerably better, as though he had slept well in a good bed rather than dozed on a stone bench after a sleepless night. But all of these facts registered as second thoughts. John's first thought, the one that had his full attention, was that the presence, the calm, sympathetic being he had met in his sleep, was still with him in the shrine. John couldn't see him or touch him, but there was no doubt at all that he was there.

John swung his legs over the side of the bench and sat up. The crick in his neck that had tortured him for months was almost gone. He sat there rubbing his eyes for a moment. The thinnest streak of gray had appeared in the sky above him. He didn't know how long he had slept. He noted all this carefully, trying to figure out if the being he felt beside him was merely another dream.

"Who are you?" he whispered. It was awkward and a little embarrassing to be speaking to the air. But the answer came immediately. It came in that same soundless, definite way I had experienced it in the hospital, when Grendel and his fans had assembled in my room.

"I'm Adam," said the being.

For the first time since It All Went to Hell, John began to cry in earnest. He cried with sheer relief, with the sense that everything was going to be all right, even though he didn't know how. But mostly he cried with joy at being reunited with Adam. It had been so long since they had seen each other that John had almost forgotten what he was like.

John did not know that this was the same reaction I had had six weeks before, when I saw the tiny face on the ultrasound screen. "Oh! It's Adam!" I had thought, not even recalling until several minutes later that I didn't know anyone named Adam. Now John was faced with the same dilemma. Each of us had become privately convinced, in the weirdest possible way, that the baby we'd named Christian Jacob Beck was actually an old friend of ours who went by the name of Adam. Furthermore, each of us believed that if we mentioned this fact to anyone, including each other, we would be seen as mentally ill, seriously disreputable, and possibly dangerous. I had read a lot of books on pregnancy, including *What to Expect When You're Expecting,* and none of them covered this particular situation.

The night in the shrine was exemplary of the way Adam operates. He goes along like any other little boy, focusing on *Star Wars* and pizza, ignoring his parents most of the time. He lets us make our own mistakes. But I have a theory that there are probably a lot of times when it's hard for him to resist coming to our rescue. I'm sure that Adam, like any good teacher, understands that doing so would rob John and me of the opportunity to develop qualities, such as serenity and courage, that come naturally to him. Even so, there are times—when fear pounces on John or me and we feel too terrified to move forward—that Adam shows his hand. Then he'll look at me carefully through his small, slanted eyes and buy me a rose, or send me a message through Parrot Woman, or reach out, the way he did in the Skytram, to keep John's attention from being riveted on his fear.

I don't know the real explanation for John's experience in the shrine that cold spring morning. But I like to imagine Adam reasoning that John needed his chin pushed up a little. Even though John was perfectly safe and well supported, the safety and support were invisible to him. His sense that his life was falling apart was no less frightening for being an illusion. I think Adam wanted to help discredit that illusion. He didn't just distract John from the terror of looking down but let him briefly touch that invisible floor, to feel it, to know that it was there by his own experience, rather than mere suggestion. It would be a while before John could stand on that floor, could get up and dance on it. But what Adam did was enough. John came home.

26

⤚ Take my advice: never attend classes at Harvard when you're seven months pregnant and the baby has Down syndrome and everybody knows it. Awful doesn't even begin to describe it.

I'm not really sure how the word got out, but it did, and fast. Obviously, Professor Goatstroke found out from John. I'd told some of my own professors as well, to explain why I looked so shell-shocked and inattentive in their classes. I don't remember mentioning it to any of my fellow students. It doesn't really matter how they found out. Whatever the mechanism, by the time I pulled myself together and showed up on campus, Adam's diagnosis was definitely hot news.

I didn't learn this because people talked to me about it. They didn't. I think they would rather have died on the rack than mention it outright. I could see that they knew by their unnaturally cheerful smiles, the strange, automatic tone of their voices, the peculiar brightness of their eyes. What is it that makes us humans stop and crane our necks to get a view of catastrophe? I have gawked at my own share of traffic accidents and disaster scenes. They fascinate me, just as they do most people, and it bothers me that I don't know why. Maybe when I gaze at a hurt human being I'm trying to take in the idea of my own fragility, or perhaps I'm glad to see that some sort of trauma has passed me by. Whatever the reason, I am quite familiar with the feeling that made my Harvard acquaintances stare at my ponderous abdomen as though it were a particularly exotic and unnerving insect they'd found under a rock.

By sheer coincidence, my Sociology of Gender seminar (the one in which I had so dramatically fainted earlier that year) had scheduled a session called "The New Obstetrical Technologies" the very week I found out about Adam's diagnosis. I skipped that class, but the next week, when I returned, the debate was still raging. The class consisted of twenty or so graduate students, who sat around a large table and discussed the weekly topic in typical seminar style. I can't tell you how surreal it felt to sit there, with Adam dancing around my interior, while my classmates argued about precisely the kind of highly unusual situation I was facing.

Most of the students in the class seemed glad that the New Obstetrical Technologies existed but were somewhat ambivalent about their moral, psychological, and social repercussions. This was pretty much how I'd always felt. However, there were other people in the class who energetically voiced opinions that hit me like a truck. I particularly remember one man leaning across the table and declaring, "It is the *duty* of every woman to screen her pregnancies and eliminate fetuses that would be a detriment to society!"

At the time, I was too stunned and exhausted to do anything more than numb out. To this day I have no idea whether that particular classmate knew about my situation. I don't even remember the guy's name. But I still think about him. I thought about him when I read an exposé of a Harvard-trained Latin American dictator who tortured and killed thousands of political opponents. I thought about him when we all discovered that the infamous Unabomber was a Harvard man as well—a genius, by all accounts.

I also thought about that seminar classmate on Adam's ninth birthday. Adam had insisted on going to a pizza-and-games arcade for his party. The only person he'd invited besides his sisters was someone I'll call Lonnie, whom Adam claimed to be his girlfriend. Although I had often heard Adam sing about Lonnie, I had never met her, or seen Adam interact with any girl. I was afraid that he would start humping her leg the second she came in range. These were fears I'd sustained since before he was born; I thought all people with Down syndrome were grossly overaffectionate. I was grossly wrong.

Lonnie turned out to be a beautiful child who had a perfectly normal brain but had been emotionally damaged by an abusive relative during the first few years of her life. She appeared timid and wary in the crowded pizza parlor until Adam rushed to stand beside her. The moment she saw him, she relaxed and broke into a shy grin. Adam had donned his best suit and tie for the occasion. He graciously took Lonnie's elbow and guided her through the pizza parlor, clearing the way in front of her with his other hand, like a cross between a professional bodyguard and the Disney version of Cinderella's prince. Lonnie's father had warned me that the rides would frighten her, and that she would probably refuse to go on them. To everyone's surprise, though, Lonnie seemed completely unafraid as long as Adam was beside her. I will never forget watching the two of them on the miniature roller coaster, Adam's hand resting reassuringly on Lonnie's arm, their faces transported with identical, absolute joy.

Now then. If my unknown classmate from the Harvard gender seminar of 1988 is anywhere out there, I'd like to speak to him directly. I'd like to ask him to put Adam on one side of the "screening" scale and the Unabomber on the other, and then tell me who is the "detriment to society." If the brilliant bomber wins out, I can only wonder, sir, exactly what kind of society you are trying to create.

The whole semester was filled with encounters like that. A couple of weeks after the New Obstetrical Technologies debate, I got into a pitched argument with a famous feminist who was visiting from Europe. I questioned her stated belief that women have babies solely to buy economic security from patriarchal power structures. I disagreed. I had to; I couldn't stop thinking about all the bizarre and intangible reasons I was having Adam.

My argument was weak and, by Harvard standards, insupportable. In any ordinary circumstances, the whole group in the seminar room would have sided with the famous feminist in wiping the intellectual floor with me. However, my classmates—all of whom, by that time, knew exactly what I was going through—felt so awkward that they just sat there, their eyes going back and forth between me and the famous feminist as though we were playing Ping-Pong. I felt a bit queasy about it, but at least I knew exactly what was happening. It made the famous feminist very nervous.

The only person at Harvard who came right up and talked to me about my predicament was one of the other teaching fellows from the Caribbean Society class. She called me a week after the diagnosis and told me that a relative of hers had committed suicide. The immense pain she was feeling seemed to level the ground between us, so that she could suddenly talk to me in a very normal and helpful way about my own fear and grief. She put me in touch with a social worker who was full of genuinely helpful information. She brought beautiful gifts for Katie and the new baby. Since then, I am always perversely happy to hear that a friend has been knocked upside the head by some unpleasant event. I am not glad they've experienced pain, but I am profoundly grateful for the down-to-earth compassion that emerges only when people face their pain and absorb it into the fabric of their lives. (This, by the way, does not mean that I myself want to go through any more pain, of any kind, ever.)

Aside from the Harvard community, there were other people around Cambridge who heard about my story and popped up out of nowhere to get a piece of the action. One woman whom I barely knew, the wife of a graduate student, started calling me every time something bad happened to her, because it made her feel better to know that my situation was more dire than hers. She actually told me this. Once she called me because her washing machine broke. She literally said, "But it's not nearly as bad as having a deformed baby, is it?" Someone else, a friend of a friend, called to assure me that a child with Down syndrome was "better than the best dog." This has certainly proven true. I wish I could say the same about the person who relayed that piece of consolation.

The people who bothered me most were the ones who wanted to make me a poster girl for the pro-life movement. Now, I have to say very clearly, right up front, that most of these were very nice people. Aside from a few political differences, I got along with them just fine. Some, though, were so pathologically invested in their cause that they didn't seem to take in anything I said. They'd be halfway through planning my participation in some form of right-wing activism before they even heard me say I disagreed with them.

I always found the ideas of this far-right group damned peculiar. They were invariably religious folks, with a devout belief in the life of the spirit. Nothing wrong with that. I myself had suspended my disbelief in a spiritual realm and was stumbling daily over more and more evidence that my world was full of things rationalist science could not explain. But this made me feel better, not worse, about the fate of those who die young, including those who die as fetuses. Why should people who believe that life exists outside of mortal bounds be the very same people who are so obsessed with a fetus's "right to life" on this messy little planet? I was confused by the pro-life position. I still am. At times I've mentioned my confusion in lectures or in print, and on some of these occasions there were audience members with such a passionate commitment to preserving life that they threatened to kill me. I guess this should have cleared up my confusion, but it hasn't. Ah, well. Perhaps in time.

There were other people who didn't seem to hear me either. Once, after I gave a little speech to a women's club and mentioned my experience having Adam, a member of the group came up to me in the women's room. She burst into tears and said, "I wanted you to know that I had to make the same decision you did, and *I chose the wrong thing!*" She had, in other words, consented to an abortion. As I watched her face contort with anguish, I felt that my heart was being ripped from its moorings. I don't know if she took in what I said, so I want to say it again, in case she's out there.

There's a Chinese word that means "soul sister," and that is the word I would use to address you in my heart. Listen to me, soul sister: Fate or luck or destiny already put you through hell once. Please don't make it worse by condemning yourself. There is no choice that would have left you feeling no guilt. Every time I watch Adam struggle to speak, every time I see another child laugh and point at him, every time I watch his face fall as he realizes he is not going to be treated like the other kids, I feel wrenched by guilt just as you did when you heard my story. Life is hard. We make the best choices we can. Condemnation, whether it comes from around you or inside you, only robs the world of another dram of compassion. God knows, we need all the compassion we can get. If you promise to try to forgive yourself, I'll try to forgive myself as well. I think, in my heart of hearts, that there is nothing for either one of us to forgive.

If I were to go on like this, to speak back to every one whose personal philosophy rode Adam's coattails into my life, this book would be way too long. Believe me, it was hard to listen to all the verbiage generated by people who heard about Adam's disability and my choice. I never thought of the right thing to say back to any of them until long after they had gone away. I did, at long last, realize that it didn't really matter what anyone else's opinion of my decision might be. What mattered was that I had made a choice that felt as though, in the end, it would bring me to the place I needed to go.

This became especially clear to me during one of John's trips to Asia, the trip from which he had decided never to return. Ever since it had become evident I wasn't in physical shape to handle John's absences alone, I'd been shuttling off to visit various family members during his trips as my own academic schedule permitted. Two weeks after the diagnosis, when John headed for Singapore, I went back to my parents' home in Utah. I carried Katie, Adam, an overnight bag, and a lot of apprehension.

My family of origin was extremely supportive during the last few months of that pregnancy. My three sisters were wonderful, calling me frequently to offer comforting advice or just to listen. My sister-in-law (the nurse) wrote me a letter so sweet it still moves me every time I see it in my files. Her husband, my eldest brother, was kind and protective in the best fraternal way. My mother did everything she could to help me feel better, but the truth was she had enough trouble dealing with Adam's condition herself, and found it almost unbearable to hear about the depth of my own sadness.

That trip to Utah, though, was the first time I would actually face anyone in my family knowing about Adam's condition. I still hadn't spoken to my father, who had never been much for phone conversation, and I didn't know how to talk to him now that I had besmirched my family's intellectual prowess by conceiving a retarded child. Every time I ran across the phrase *mongoloid idiot*, I felt the weight of the thousands, maybe millions of times the word *idiot* had been used to disparage and dismiss people in my family's conversations. Now I was going back, bearing a medically diagnosed "idiot" in my belly. Part of me knew that no one in my family wanted to hurt me. Another part was terrified of what they might say to me, how they might act, when I was with them in the flesh.

As it turned out, they didn't say anything. I mean not one thing. My father picked Katie and me up at the airport. All the way home, about an hour's drive, he talked about some obscure text he had encountered in his research. When we arrived at my family's swimming-pool-blue estate, my mother talked to me about Katie and John and school. I'm telling you, it was bizarre. I kept thinking about Eugène Ionesco's plays, in which polite society types sit around discussing the weather, refusing to acknowledge that the people around them are on fire, or turning into rhinoceroses. Perfect strangers were calling me on the phone because they'd heard about my baby and my decision, but here, in the bosom of my natal family, nobody wanted to talk about it.

At one point I figured I'd just have to take the bull by the horns. I was sitting in my parents' living room with my mother, father, and one of my older brothers. Katie was playing on the floor amid the piles of Stuff. Someone had just said something about it's not being fair that some people have successful careers and some people don't. I saw an opening, took a deep breath, and said, "Yeah, I guess that's just how life works. It made me sad every time I saw a healthy baby boy in the airport."

Even I, who know my family well, would never have predicted their reaction. My father looked at me and began to laugh—not just a little laugh, but a loud, long, forced guffaw, as if I were a bad comedian he was trying to encourage. My brother laughed along, though not as heartily. My mother just sat there knitting. Then my father launched into a scathing attack on a local university, because he had read in the newspaper that a woman with an IQ of only 70 had managed to complete all the requirements for graduation, after ten years of diligent effort. My brother took this thread and ran with it, commenting on a news story about two retarded people who had gotten married. His position was that if this were allowed to happen, the half-brains in question should at least be voluntarily sterilized. From that point on, it was as if, no matter how hard they tried not to talk about my baby, they couldn't help it. I know they weren't consciously choosing topics that would eviscerate me right there in the living room. They were very worried about me, and meant nothing but the best. But, as I've said, denial tends to leak.

Fortunately, although this conversation left me almost completely devastated, I was, in the end, able to cope with it. This is solely because after my first year at Harvard, when I was feeling a tiny bit down and spent most of my time comparison shopping for the quickest and most painless method of suicide, I had gone into therapy. On my first visit, the psychologist asked me some questions about my family, which I answered honestly, not suspecting that our gang was much different from anybody else. Then he asked me how many siblings I had. I'd told him already—seven—but I repeated it.

"Holy mackerel!" he shouted jubilantly. "I'm gonna cash in on this one!"

I think he gave me most of my therapy free.

➔ I'd been in Utah a few days when one of my cousins came to visit me. Lydia is almost exactly my age, and by the time we were both in our mid-twenties she'd had enough troubles of her own to satisfy your average small city. When she showed up at the house, my parents and brother had reverted to avoiding any overt comment on my situation. I told Lydia about it, and mentioned that it was making me a little uncomfortable, sort of like having an armed nuclear warhead under my bed. Lydia pointed out to me that our fathers (who were brothers) had only one way of expressing emotion, and that was laughter. They had passed this imperative on to their children. Need to scream? Scream with laughter. Need to cry? Shed tears of mirth. Need to pretend that someone's baby isn't disabled? Have yourself a good haw-haw-haw. Works for any occasion.

Paradoxically, Lydia was also the one who first helped me use that double-edged gift of humor to cope with having Adam. We were out in her car, cruising through the snow-covered mountains that had always soothed me so much, with Katie strapped into the backseat and Adam bulging out toward the dashboard. Lydia asked a string of thoughtful questions. We talked about how she had felt during some of her own life crises, especially the early death of her father. We got a little weepy. At one point Lydia pulled over and stopped the car, parking it near a snowbank until we'd both cried ourselves out. Then she sat up straight, wiped her nose, and sighed.

"Look," she said. "Here's what's going to happen. You're going to have one really smart kid, and one really dumb kid. Is that so bad?"

I found myself laughing—not the way my father had laughed, but truly and spontaneously. That kind of laughter doesn't drive tears away. It complements them.

"No, I guess it isn't so bad," I said. Then I bit my lip. "It's just so hard to think about the way people will look at him. At me."

I had read about this in several books by parents of disabled kids. They all agreed that one of the challenges of having a child with Down syndrome is learning to bear the shame of being a public spectacle.

"Okay, so let's imagine the worst," said Lydia. "You're sitting somewhere—at the bus stop, wherever—and you've got your baby, like this." She pantomimed holding a little bundle on her lap. "Then some fat, middle-aged woman with bad teeth comes over to you and says, 'Hey, you! Looks to me like there's something wrong with that there baby!' "

I shuddered. "Exactly," I said.

"Well, here's what you do," said Lydia. She looked intently at the face of the invisible baby. Then her eyes widened in horror. "Oh, my *God*!" she shouted. *"You're right!"*

We dissolved, both of us. I laughed so hard that all my overstretched abdominal muscles went into a severe cramp, and I had to get out and walk around the car.

After that conversation with my cousin, it was a lot easier to tolerate the strange, determined way some of my other relatives were avoiding talking to me about the baby. Nevertheless, three days before I left Utah, I finally broke down. I had been to the local mall, buying clothes for Katie. For some reason, seeing the throngs of little boys in the children's clothing store had made my heart ache so intensely I could hardly even drive. I wept all the way to my parents' house, and when I got there I couldn't stop. My father was there, reading a book, when I walked in.

"What's all this?" he said, in a jocular tone. "What's all this?"

"I'm sorry," I sobbed. "I'm sorry, Daddy. This is just so hard for me."

My poor father. He fell completely apart. I have never seen any grown man cry the way my father cried that day. The man was more Harvard than Harvard: almost eighty years old, white-haired, dignified, the very archetype of the eccentric professorial genius. But he sobbed like a five-year-old with a broken heart.

There was no question of his trying to comfort me; I could sense that immediately. You can feel it when another person's despair is deeper than your own. Now that my father wasn't hiding behind his social mask, it was clear to me that he was far less equipped to cope with my situation than I was myself. And besides, I had help. In the honesty of that moment, I could feel the invisible helpers ranged around me, surrounding me with empathy and concern. Now that I had stopped disbelieving in them, they were almost as tangible as my father. I knew they were there for him, too. But he couldn't see them. He couldn't feel them.

I looked at my weeping parent the way I had looked at Dr. Grendel when he had brought his fear into the infirmary at University Health Services. I did not see the imposing, powerful father of my childhood. I saw an old man who had never, not for one moment of his life, believed that it was possible to be loved for himself. A man who had been raised to be a genius the way a Nazi is raised to be a bigot, who had been judged at every stage of his life by intelligence tests, advanced degrees, and the rigors of academia. His intellectual brilliance was the single barrier that kept back the utter barrenness of a life without love or belonging.

Or so he thought. It wasn't true. I knew it wasn't, because I loved him. But ever since I was a teenager in therapy, I had known that all the love I felt for my father would never make it through his defenses to be felt and understood. Now, hearing him sob so hard he could barely breathe, I knew he still couldn't feel my love, lost as it was in the deluge of his own pain. At least I realized I wasn't the only one working on it. I could feel love radiating to my father from the invisible people around us, from every corner of that Stuff-encrusted room, from every corner of the swimming-pool-blue house, from all the space around us in every direction. It was there for my father as it was there for me, for Adam, for Katie, for Lydia, for every one of us.

I found myself hoping, all over again, my childhood hope that somehow, something would get through to my father's heart before he died. I wanted desperately for him to feel the inconceivable comfort of knowing that, brilliant or dull, genius or idiot, he was and always had been essentially and unalterably lovable. From my new perspective, the one I had picked up while expecting Adam, I hoped the Bunraku puppeteers had a plan for how this might be done. It seemed likely that they did—but on the other hand, I knew that my father was as tough-minded and terrified a soul as the puppeteers were likely to encounter. I couldn't imagine any strategy to break through his defenses. But what the hell, I thought, maybe they'd figure out something that would work for him.

After all, they'd figured out something for me.

27

⤵ When John and I were reunited in Cambridge after the March trip, we weren't exactly sure how to talk to each other. Both of us had changed a lot in the short time we'd been apart. We each felt as vulnerable as a chick fresh out of the egg, stumbling around in our new personalities with our feathers wet and our legs all wobbly. We hadn't talked explicitly about the shift of perspective that was happening inside each of us; we both feared being misunderstood, even ridiculed, if we revealed how confused and how tender we were under the skin. So we hid ourselves from each other in a delicate and awkward wordlessness. Actually, I believe this is pretty much what a lot of people do most of the time.

The bulk of our conversations consisted of my conveying to John the latest information I had read about Down syndrome. I believed that if I could learn everything about the condition, I'd be able to predict what our lives with Adam would be like. Instead, everything I learned intensified the feeling that our future, and the future of our child, was almost completely up for grabs. To begin with, Adam had about a 60 percent chance of living through his birth. After that there were other percentages: 40 percent chance of a serious heart defect, 30 percent chance of kidney failure, 26 percent chance of respiratory difficulty, and so on. And on. Talking about actual problems is a wonderful way to move forward through shock and grief to acceptance. But talking about uncertainty can't lead anywhere but back to uncertainty—and it is a painful journey.

The more we realized this, the less John and I talked. We kept up pragmatic, necessary discussions about our daily schedules, Katie's care and feeding, my medical appointments. John's family socialization as a *mono* person, someone whose entire conversational repertoire focused on physical objects, came in mighty handy at this point.

Still, there were wordless ways in which John and I managed to connect during those difficult weeks. One of these was nitpicking. You may have heard this term used to mean petty criticism, but I mean it liter-ally. We didn't say a word. We just picked nits. To understand this, you must learn a few charming details about our insect friend the louse. As a child I had picked up the impression that lice were large, beetlelike crea-tures who built major establishments, similar to termite hills, in the wigs of Baroque Europeans. Actually, they are tiny little things (the lice, not the Europeans). They're so small you don't usually realize right away that they're living on your head. Ordinary shampooing doesn't kill them or wash them away; in fact, they seem to love it. And while our little buddies are frolicking between the roots of human hair, they lay itsy-bitsy eggs, which they anchor to individual hair shafts. The eggs are called nits. Yanking them out of your hair is the literal meaning of the verb *to nitpick.*

I know this is disgusting. It's not like I love to go around talking about it. I'm not sure I've ever admitted it before, even to close friends. It's just that to fully understand the condition John and I reached when we were expecting Adam, you have to know that nitpicking was—honest to God—one of the most enjoyable things we shared during that time. I'm no marriage counselor, but it seems to me that when a lice infestation becomes the high point of your relationship, things have gone seriously awry.

The first time John brought lousy associates home from Singapore, way back in October, we did everything short of sandblasting our apart-ment and everything in it, especially our heads. I'd read that hair dye can damage a fetus if the mother uses it during her first trimester of preg-nancy, and it crossed my mind that the antilouse shampoo we picked up from the pharmacy might have similar effects. I didn't give a rat's ass. I rubbed that stuff all over my body, and left it there until I was afraid my hair would fall right out. John, needless to say, was engaged in similar pursuits. For a time, we were sure the lice were dead and gone. But six weeks later, I felt an all-too-familiar itch on my scalp, and we both went through the entire delousing project yet again. Katie never did get them, but John and I had to sustain this on-and-off battle until nearly the time Adam was born.

Anyway, after nuking the lice with the special shampoo, one is left with the tiny dead nits still stuck to one's hair. The antilouse shampoo is sold with a little comb, which is supposed to remove the nits, but it doesn't work. The only way you can really get rid of the little bastards is to pick through your hair with your fingernails. This became an obsessive habit for John and me. People who knew us at the time probably remember us with our hands constantly twitching toward our heads, like Son of Sam when the invisible dog was talking to him.

This is a great hobby, as far as it goes, but you always have the disadvantage of not being able to *see* the nits in your own hair. I don't know when John and I started taking turns holding each other's heads in our laps and going through each other's hair with intense concentration, like a couple of baboons. I do know that it was really soothing. It made me think of something I'd learned in Folklore and Mythology 100, which I took as an undergraduate (this course, arguably the least challenging class at Harvard, was informally known as FM 100: Easy Listening). In all the Nordic sagas, you see, after the hero had gone through some epic travail, he would be washed and *deloused* by the heroine. At the time I read this, I thought it unutterably revolting. Now it makes me a bit nostalgic.

The other form of communication that held our relationship together during that pregnancy centered on the little plastic alphabet letters that we had bought for Katie, the ones that stuck to our refrigerator door with magnets. Katie liked them a lot, although she didn't seem particularly interested in learning to read. Mostly, she peeled them off the refrigerator, chewed on them for a while, and then flushed them down the toilet. We lost many letters in this manner, and John kept doggedly buying whole new alphabets, as though he could move Katie to literacy by sheer persistence.

At one point, our fridge was left with an odd and limited assortment of letters, specifically (in alphabetical order), E, F, L, M, N, O, and U. I know the exact letters because one day I went into the kitchen and discovered that they had been arranged to spell the phrase "MOLE FUN." I stood there looking at the refrigerator, rearranged the letters to spell "FOUL MEN," and left. The next day, I found the letter "W" in Katie's crib. I soon had the words "MENU FLOW" up on the fridge. Later, after John had been there, it said "FUN LAME SOW" (he'd gotten lucky and found A and S somewhere in Katie's room).

This went on for weeks. We never, ever discussed it, but we kept silently upping the ante by adding new letters we found between the sofa cushions and under the bed and behind the books on the shelves. Over time, we developed unspoken rules: at first, for example, we would invert letters like M and W to get more mileage out of the selection, but this quickly came to be considered a cheap solution. Then there were random combinations of unrelated words, but gradually it became clear that a really diligent rearranger could always create a cogent thought unit out of the available letters.

By the time we had found all the letters that remained in the apartment, we ended up with a combination that could be rearranged to form such thought-provoking phrases as "MANGY SULPHUR COW FUEL" or "LU, SPEW FANCY GHOUL RUM" or "WHY GUMS FOR UNCLE PAUL?" For me, the high point of this game occurred on the day when, after half an hour of hard thinking in front of the refrigerator, I realized that the letters before me could spell out "WALL OF GRUMPY EU-NUCHS." It was a major epiphany. I looked at my creation with almost sublime joy. I could tell John was impressed, too, because although he never mentioned it, he left the phrase untouched for several days. The image of that wall, of all those eunuchs crammed together, five deep, three high, bitching at each other, remains vivid in my mind's eye to this day. It is one of the creative fruits that emerged from the pain and suffering we went through while expecting Adam. Sweet are the uses of adversity.

⟜ March was almost over before John and I broke through our mutual silence. I awoke from a fitful sleep at about three o'clock on a Sunday morning, when Adam socked me in the ribs. I had been waking up regularly around this time, and it was not fun. No matter how hard I tried to think positively and keep my chin up, no matter how much I reminded

myself that many people had been through far worse and come out in-
tact, all the most frightening things I had learned about Down syndrome
floated into my mind in the predawn gloom, paralyzing me with dread
of both the known and the unknown.

After brooding for a while, I heaved my ripening self off the stress
mat and plodded down the hall toward the kitchen. Perhaps, I thought,
a slab of steak would help. Once I got there and flipped on the kitchen
light, my attention wandered away from food and toward the fridge letters, which now read "WHELP YOUR FUNGAL SCUM." I was busy re-
arranging them when a shadowy shape loomed out of the darkness. I
gave a sharp yip of surprise and terror before I realized that it was John.

"Don't *do* that!" I said.

John grinned wearily. He looked hammered. His eyes had sunk so far
back from fatigue that they were almost completely hidden in the
shadow of his brows.

"Gotcha," he said.

"It's not funny, John." I was in no mood for levity.

"What are you doing up?" he said.

"Couldn't sleep," I replied. "What are *you* doing?"

"Hungry," he said. "And I might as well start changing my body clock
now."

I nodded.

"I want chocolate chip cookies," said John.

My mood brightened a little. We are both very big on chocolate
chip cookies, John and I. It was one of the major things that brought us
together. The previous year, when we had to walk more than ten miles
in the cold on an average day, we had baked and snarfed down close
to our weight in chocolate chip cookies every week or so. Since Adam
was conceived, however, my cookie consumption had fallen to nil, and
John didn't like to indulge alone—that, as we all know, is one of the
warning signs of addiction.

Now, after months of abstinence, John was opening cupboards,
pulling out the familiar ingredients, lining them up on the counter. I felt
an echo of the festive tone that had always accompanied our cookie-

baking episodes. I waddled over to the one chair that fit in our tiny kitchen and sat down to watch.

"How are you feeling?" asked John politely, as he pulled out a mixing bowl.

"Fine."

This was about as deep as our conversations had been for several weeks. As I watched John get a pound of butter out of the refrigerator and put a stick into the bowl, I managed to say, "I talked to my mom today."

"Oh?" John measured white and brown sugar into the bowl and mashed the ingredients together with a wooden spoon.

"Yeah," I said listlessly. "She met another woman with a Down syndrome grandson. The kid's fifteen. He's doing really well."

"That's nice," said John. He took the electric mixer out of its drawer and assembled it. For a truly great chocolate chip cookie, it is essential to beat the sugar and butter together very, very thoroughly.

"She said he cleans his own bedroom," I continued. "Keeps it neat as a pin."

"Great!" said John, with obviously feigned enthusiasm.

"I guess it should have cheered me up," I said, "but it didn't." I could feel tears in my eyes. I had been getting better and better at repressing my grief in front of John, but at three in the morning my emotions were hard to check.

"The thing is," I said, "I don't want a teenage son who just keeps his room as neat as a pin." My voice trembled a little. "I kept thinking while I was talking to her—people don't know how lucky they are to have a teenage son who messes up his room, and puts stupid posters on the wall, and stays out too late, and has a girlfriend, and applies to college." The tears brimmed and slid out into my eyelashes. I sniffed.

John said nothing. He turned on the mixer and stuck it into the bowl. It snarled, struggling with the cold butter. He pushed up the speed control, and the snarl rose to a high, angry whine. This was normal mixer behavior; I had seen it many times. That night, however, instead of set-tling into a healthy-sounding whir, the whine got higher and higher, louder and louder. John tried to turn the mixer off. It didn't work. The mixer screamed and flailed like a huge, tormented insect. Then there was a small *pop*, and a cloud of smoke rose from its body. It stopped whining. It was dead.

"Oh, great," said John. "Just great."

For some reason, this was just one thing too much for me. I curled up in my chair as best I could, my knees pressed against my pregnant torso, and started to cry in earnest.

John turned on me, his lips tight with annoyance. "What are you blubbering about?"

"It *broke*," I wailed.

"Yes, I realize that," John snapped. "I was holding it."

"Everything breaks," I sobbed. "Nothing goes right, everything goes wrong. Something's happened to us, John. We can't do things anymore. Not anything. I mean, how could you expect us to make a good baby when we can't even make a good cookie?"

"Oh, for crying out loud, Martha!" John's voice was getting loud. "Would you grab the reins? I'm sick and tired of hearing how miserable your life is."

I cried harder. "I'm just scared," I said.

John cracked two eggs into the mixing bowl and started whipping them into the other ingredients with the wooden spoon. He looked as though he had plenty of energy to compensate for the broken mixer.

"Scared of what?" he said. "Of a little baby who's not as perfect as you think he ought to be?" He dumped flour into the mixing bowl and began to thrash at it with the spoon. A mist of flour rose from the bowl, covering his hands and forearms.

"I didn't say I wanted him to be perfect," I said. "I just want him to be normal. That's all I want. Just normal."

"Bullshit," John barked. He measured salt and baking soda into the dough and went back to work with the mixing spoon.

I raised my dripping face out of my hands. "Excuse me?"

"That is total bullshit," he repeated. "You don't want this baby to be normal. You'd throw him in a Dumpster if he just turned out to be normal. What you really want is for him to be superhuman."

I squinted at him. "What the hell are you talking about?"

John added chocolate chips and beat them in. At this stage, of course, the dough is sticky and stiff and hard to mix. But John whipped away at it as if it were nothing but egg whites. He was starting to sweat.

"For your information," I said in my most acid tone, "I was the one who decided to keep this baby, even though he's got Down's. *You* were the one who wanted to throw him in a Dumpster."

"How would you know?" John's voice was still gaining volume. "You never asked me what I wanted, did you? No! You never even *asked* me!"

I was so stunned I stopped crying. "What is going on with you, John? I thought—"

"Yeah, that's right!" he shouted. "You thought, you thought, you thought! You thought all kinds of things, didn't you? You thought old John would just strap on the saddle and take you wherever you want to go. And then I'm supposed to feel sorry for you?"

"John—"

He went into baby talk. "Poor wittle Mawfa," he simpered. "She has to have a *bad* baby. She has to have a *freak*, instead of a *perfect* little boy like she wants."

I was staring at him with utter incredulity. "What planet are you from?" I said.

"You act like you're on some big moral pedestal," John shot back. "You think it's such a big deal to keep this baby. But I know what's really going on inside you. You don't want him. He disgusts you. The only reason you're having this baby at all is that you didn't have the guts to get an abortion."

I came out of the chair straight at him, my head low, like a bull in the ring. I had a few steps to pick up speed, and I weighed considerably more than usual. My shoulder hit John right below the rib cage, knocking him back against the counter.

John had to struggle for a minute to get his breath back. "Oh, that's good," he said. "That's just wonderful. Physically violent women make great mommies."

I wanted to kill him. All the emotion that had been hidden behind weeks of careful, civilized silence rushed from my guts into my head, my heart, my arms and legs. I felt like a tiger tearing down a trap. I wanted to rip the plumbing apart with my bare hands and beat down the walls with it. Instead, I grabbed a lump of cookie dough from the mixing bowl and pushed it into John's face.

"*How dare you talk to me like that?*" I screamed. "How *dare* you? Is there one tiny molecule somewhere in your brain that can begin to understand what this is like for me?" I thumped myself in the abdomen with both hands, so hard that I could see John wince through his mask of cookie dough. "*This is my son!*" I sobbed. "He's a part of me! If you don't want him, you can leave us both, but *he is my son,* and that's why I'm keeping him, even if he is a freak!"

"There you go!" John shouted. "You can't even mention him without calling him names, can you? No matter what he does, he'll never be good enough for you. Never!" He scraped a lump of dough off his cheek and threw it at me.

I dodged. "What the *hell* are you talking about?" I hollered. "Are you completely insane?"

"Do you know how this baby is going to feel?" John yelled. "Do you know how you're going to make him feel? Every day of his life, he's going to know he's not good enough. He's going to try and try and work and work and work and work and *work,* and it's *never going to be enough for you!*"

He seized another piece of dough from the bowl and slung it at me. I turned my head at the last second, and it hit me just above the ear, clinging to my hair like a misshapen barrette.

"*Why can't he ever be enough for you?*" John was still yelling. Another lump of dough whizzed by me and stuck to the wall.

"*Why does he have to work so hard?*" This one hit me in the arm.

"*How come he has to be perfect, and do everything just right, and never make a mistake?"* Another dough ball landed on my shoulder and stuck to my bathrobe.

"John," I said, in a low, dangerous voice. "John, calm down."

"Why can't you just love him because he's a little boy?" John screamed as a final projectile missed me and landed in the sink. *"Why can't you love him as he is?"*

His voice had degenerated into a hoarse sob, and tears were running in two steady streams over the cookie dough on his face. John touched his cheek and brought his hand away slowly, staring at it in amazement.

"There's water on my face," he said in a baffled whisper. He looked at me with complete bewilderment. "How come there's water on my face?"

I don't think John had cried in front of another person since he could remember. I looked at him, and the anger seemed to drain out of me all at once, leaving me scoured and exhausted.

"Honey," I said, in my normal speaking voice, "you realize that you're not really talking about the baby, don't you? You're talking about yourself."

John nodded.

"Do you also realize that you're not really talking to me?"

He raised his eyes to mine and looked into them almost desperately. "I'm not?" he whispered.

"No." I moved forward and wiped some of the dough off his cheek. "Listen to me," I said. "I'm not your mom, and I'm not your dad, and I'm not your church, and I'm not Harvard. Actually, I'm not much of anything. But for what it's worth, I love you as you are. I thought you knew that."

John's dough-smeared face crumpled, and for the first time ever, I saw him really cry. It seemed that all the men in my life were doing it.

I put my arms around him. "Come here," I said. I led him into the living room, pushed him gently down on the sofa. John was as docile as he had been angry. I sat down next to him. The sliding glass door that led out to our tiny balcony admitted a faint golden shimmer from the halogen streetlights along Massachusetts Avenue. All of Harvard was laid out below us, the spires of its chapels and dormitories stabbing up like dark blades against the dull reflected glow of the low-hanging clouds.

We sat awhile without saying anything. John cried for several minutes, the kind of healing cry that most women know well, and most men never allow themselves. I, for once, was not crying. I sat with my arm around my husband, our sides pressed together so that when Adam kicked, we both felt it. After a while, John became quiet again. But it wasn't the volatile, brittle, repressed silence that we'd kept for the past few weeks. It was the calm that comes when all the dirty truths have finally been spoken.

"I thought I would be the only one who could love him," John said finally.

"Me too," I said.

John reached over and pulled some of the cookie dough out of my hair. "You're different than I remember you."

"So are you."

He took a long, deep breath and stretched his arms to the ceiling, bringing one down around my shoulders. "You still scared?" he said.

"Yeah."

"So am I."

We sat with that one for a while. We could hear the subway trains rumbling by under Mass Ave. When they passed the sidewalk grilles, a brilliant flash of blue light would briefly gleam and then disappear. Three trains went by before we spoke again.

"I have to tell you something," said John. He sounded very serious, a little nervous. I felt my heart speed up, anticipating at least a thousand terrible things. I was getting very good at this way of thinking.

"I don't want you to take this the wrong way," said John slowly, "but I . . . I don't want to name him Chris."

I blinked. "You don't?"

"It's not what you think," said John. "It's not that I wouldn't want him to have the family name or anything, and it isn't that I feel different about him now that we know about . . ." His voice trailed off.

"Okay," I said cautiously.

"It's just that it doesn't seem like the right name," said John. "I don't know how to explain it, but it just doesn't."

My scalp was beginning to prickle, and it wasn't lice. It was the familiar electrical charge that seemed to run through my body more and more often. It had reached the point where I felt it every time I even thought about the baby—about Adam. That was what I called him in my mind, now, all the time. The name had pressed so insistently against my brain that I had finally just surrendered to it, wondering what I was going to say to John when it came time to fill out the birth certificate. Or the death certificate.

"Are you upset?" John's worried eyes were studying my face.

"No, no," I said. "I . . . actually, I agree. I don't think Chris sounds right for him." I remembered the ultrasound clinic, the familiar little person on the screen waving at me like an old friend.

"What do you want to name him?" I asked John.

He sighed and scraped some of the dough off his face with his fingernail. "I think his name is Adam."

The baby did a somersault. We both felt it. I looked at my husband, wide-eyed, and my entire body began to tingle as though I had been plugged into a socket.

"John," I said, "we have to talk."

28

⌐ Adam was seven when my cousin Lydia and her sister Sylvia talked me into visiting a psychic. I'd never done it before, and don't really intend to do it again, but my cousins convinced me that until I'd gone in for a reading, I simply hadn't been on all the rides.

The psychic wasn't at all what I'd expected. She was an eminently normal-looking woman in her mid-thirties, who lived in Magna, Utah. Whenever I tell this story, I always get the same question: "If she was really psychic, why was she living in Magna, Utah?" You will agree that this is a good question, especially if you've ever been to Magna. Not being psychic myself, I don't have the answer. I suppose it will have to remain a Blessed Mystery.

At any rate, I showed up at the psychic's place of business with my mind as open as I could get it. I'd been trying hard to live by my new credo, in which anything must be considered possible until it is proven false. Still, I expected the woman to say things like, "Someone you once knew died in the last ten years, of a heart attack or cancer or some other disease, or possibly an accident. Or maybe you didn't actually *know* this person, but you knew *of* him. Or her."

Instead, the psychic parked herself in an easy chair across from me and closed her eyes for about fifteen minutes. Then, eyes still shut, she gave me a detailed description of my life. She included things I was positive my cousin couldn't have known, such as the nature of this bladder disease I have, which is too embarrassing to mention to anyone, although I have now announced it in print. I guess the secret's out anyway, because this psychic knew all about it.

I have to admit, I was impressed.

I was so busy being skeptical that I didn't do the logical thing, which was to ask the psychic about stock investments. Instead, I had her describe other people I knew. I'd give her the name and approximate age of each person. She'd sit there for a while with her eyes closed, and then tell me about them. In detail. I threw everything I could at her, to see how good she really was. I asked her about people I'd met in Japan, in Switzerland, in deepest Communist China. I'm telling you, she was good. There was no fumbling around. She knew who had lost a finger in a factory accident, who had just gone to work for a bank, who had been divorced and remarried within three weeks. Nothing she said had any implications for my life, but I enjoyed just sitting there seeing what she could do. It was like watching a contortionist: not particularly useful, but most amazing.

Toward the end of the sitting, I asked the psychic about my children. I gave her their names and birth dates, starting with Katie. She told me everything I already knew about Katie's sensitive personality, her childhood bouts with ear infections, her insistence on never being late, and her love of Baroque choral music, which seemed to spring with her from the womb. Cool, I thought.

Then I gave the psychic Adam's name and birthday. She sat there for a while, as usual, with her eyes closed. Then she said, "Adam isn't like your other children."

I said nothing. I was careful not to change my expression, in case she was peeking.

"I have to explain this to you," said the psychic. "You see, Adam is an angel."

I felt a little bristly around the collar, but I still didn't move.

"Angels are different from other metaphysical beings," she went on. "Occasionally they decide to incarnate—to become human for a while. Not that they have to, you understand. Sometimes that's just the best way to do what they want to do."

The psychic then went into a quasi-technical and very wacky-sounding New Age theological discussion, which I found difficult to follow and even more difficult to swallow. I tried to take it in without rolling my eyes, but it was a struggle. After about ten minutes or so, the lecture wound down.

I cleared my throat. "Adam has Down syndrome," I said.

The psychic didn't seem at all surprised. She just shrugged.

"That," she said, "has nothing to do with it."

This was what clinched my belief in her psychic gifts. If she had said, "Oh, yes, that makes it perfectly clear; *all* our little retarded brothers and sisters are angels," I would have looked upon her with a more jaundiced eye. I've heard that line many, many times, from people so sanctimoniously sweet that just standing near them will rot your teeth. These are the same people who always tell me that God would never give *them* such a child, because they are too weak to be deserving. They are the people who look at Adam and then tell me, in a stage whisper, "Mongoloids are always so content, aren't they?" I wish these "contented-mongoloid" theorists had to deal with Adam when he's sleep deprived or his dad is out of town or his sisters are picking on him. It's true he doesn't indulge in the sort of morose weeping to which I am prone. Mostly he dismantles the furniture. But there are definitely times when he is not content.

At any rate, the Magna psychic did not come back at me with any of the hundred clichés I'd heard targeted at people with Down syndrome. She didn't even want to talk about genetic disabilities. She wanted to talk about angels.

"Anyone you meet could be an angel," she said. "Usually you just see them in passing—they show up to do something and then discarnate again. But sometimes they come the regular way, as babies, and live like other humans for a lifetime. Like your son. I'd imagine a few of them have Down syndrome, but I don't know. It's an interesting question."

By this time I was squinting at her out of one eye and contemplating whether I should ask her about what research methodology she had used to get all this information on angels. Then I remembered that, without any research beyond sitting quietly, she had just accurately described almost everyone I knew. I decided to leave the question alone.

Of course, just because I believe that the Magna psychic had a gift of some sort doesn't mean I buy into her theology wholesale. Been there, done that. I saw a bumper sticker once that said, "My karma ran over my dogma," which pretty much sums up my feelings about most religious cosmologies. (Ironically, it was after Adam was born, when I began to believe in God, that I explicitly left the religion of my childhood.)

Given the eclectic and constantly shifting nature of my metaphysical inclinations, I will probably never feel certain exactly what an angel is. The Magna psychic could have been 100 percent right, all the way down the line. Or maybe the ancient Chinese were on to something, and we're all haunted by numberless ancestors. Or maybe Catholic saints. Or leprechauns. Hey, I'll go there.

One thing I don't believe, though, is that there are *no* spiritual beings around us. They popped into my awareness often enough while I was expecting Adam to disprove that hypothesis to my satisfaction. I don't know what to call them, I don't know how they work. But I know they're there.

I have consciously believed this ever since the night that John and I sat on our couch, looking out over Harvard Square, and told each other everything. I told him about the invisible hands that rescued me when I was caught in the smoke and, later, when I was bleeding. He told me about the "dream—sort of" that he'd had in Japan. I told him about the Seeing Thing. We talked about the way Dr. Grendel's face had floated around in two parts as he sat on my hospital bed. We went over all the strange coincidences that kept occurring, like the way Sibyl just *happened* to show up with exactly the groceries I craved exactly when I needed them, and later just *happened* to know every little, tiny detail one could ever hope to know about infants with birth defects. As far as I was concerned, Sibyl alone constituted a major miracle. John had to agree.

We didn't sleep at all that night. We talked, and talked, and paced around, and talked, and baked what was left of the cookie dough, and talked some more. Our immense physical fatigue was more than offset by an intoxicating sense of freedom, as we both learned that we could talk to each other about our bizarre new beliefs, and be believed. More than just companionship, we found validation in each other's experiences. It is one thing to suspect, in your own fevered mind, that all kinds of supernatural things are happening to you. It is quite another to hear that someone else's fevered mind has its own suspicions, and that your experiences complement each other like two halves of a broken seal. Reality has never felt quite so surreal as it did to me that night. I had to keep drawing in big gulps of air, as if I were sprinting to keep up with the pace at which my worldview was being transformed.

One of the things we talked about that night was the name Adam. We tried to remember if we'd discussed that name during some half-remembered conversation early in my pregnancy, but we honestly didn't think we had. We'd both simply felt an overpowering sense, not only of rightness but of *recognition,* when the name and the baby came together. I had felt it at the ultrasound clinic, John in the Japanese shrine, but both of us had the sense that Adam had been Adam since long before then. It felt as though we had known him by that name for years and years and years. Forever.

I still don't know if there's any compelling metaphysical reason for Adam's name, but I know that it carries a lot of meaning. We looked it up that night, and found that *Adam* is an Aramaic word meaning "man of earth." The name reflects an ancient belief that God made the original man from mud, before breathing life into him.

This aspect of Adam's name wouldn't really come home to me until a few months after he was born. I was standing in line at an airport when an old, very decrepit-looking woman went past in a wheelchair, pushed by an airline attendant. Suddenly, the woman slumped forward and pitched to the floor. The attendant tried to pick her up. When he couldn't, he ran desperately for help. It didn't arrive in time. While the attendant was gone, before I could even look away, the woman died. It was the first human death I had ever witnessed, and it was very strange. Nothing about her was visibly altered at the moment of her death; it's just that one instant there was an old woman on the floor, and the next, there was only a body. You could feel it. Whether she went into oblivion or eternal life, I don't know, but she was gone. The body, without her in it, truly seemed to be nothing but clay. I think about that sometimes, about the fact that the part of Adam I see with my eyes—his round little face, his disproportionate limbs, his unsteady gait—is only a sort of housing, a compilation of carefully organized chemicals animated by some force that no one can really explain. It is only a "man of earth."

Then there is the fact that the name Adam can be taken to mean

Everyman, the whole species of us. The first time I changed Adam's diaper, when he was stretched out in the hospital bassinet, as scrawny and naked and vulnerable as a bug without its shell, I thought that he pretty much exemplified the human condition. I remembered a quote from *King Lear*, one that had always stuck in my mind although I'd made no conscious attempt to memorize it. I said it to Adam. "Thou art the thing itself," I told him. "Unaccommodated man is no more but such a poor, bare, forked animal as thou art." Adam turned his delicate, fuzzy-peach head to look at my face and snuffled a bit through his nose.

It was our first real conversation.

Then, too, the name Adam reminds me of the Fall, that multifaceted legend of human separation from some native spiritual realm, and the mortality that is supposed to take us back to it. It reminds me that we are born innocent but ignorant, and that to remedy the second of these conditions we inevitably surrender the first. The word *Adam* has been used to signify a great many things to members of my culture. Every time I call my son for dinner, I am reminded of them all. I like that. I like it a lot.

John and I spent a lot of time wondering about meanings that first night we sat up and told each other the naked truth. We came up with many interpretations of the Adam situation and everything connected to it. I'm pretty sure they were all wrong, or at the very least much too simplistic. The most important thing about that conversation was not any dramatic conclusion we drew from our experiences over the preceding few months but the fact that those experiences supported each other. For the first time, this made them harder for me to dismiss than to believe.

The next day I dropped Katie off at day care and set off for class as usual. I never got there. I was too stunned, too full of wonder, to sit still. I kept walking around Harvard, staring at the familiar buildings, the familiar people, as though I had just climbed off a spacecraft from Neptune. The whole universe seemed different to me. I didn't know how to be at Harvard while believing such irrational things. I went into the Science Center, a huge, cold, concrete structure designed to resemble a Polaroid camera (Edwin Land, the photographic inventor, donated the money for the building). The people in the Science Center cafeteria were chatting and smoking and slugging back industrial-strength coffee as usual, just as if there weren't angels all over the place.

Part of me wanted to run up to everyone I saw and shake them all by the collar, shouting, *"Yo! Listen! We are not alone!"* right into their ears until they really heard me. The other part of me knew damn well that if I so much as whispered what I was thinking, these people would set about destroying me in a manner similar to the Chinese "death of a thousand cuts," in which bystanders are encouraged to slice off bits and pieces of a prisoner until he expires. Of course they'd use words instead of bamboo knives, but the psychological effect would be similar. I kept darting my eyes around, wondering if people could sense that I had moved into a world where rationalism was a necessary but insufficient explanation for what I experienced. Some people did look at me rather strangely, but I think it was just because any woman at that stage of pregnancy walks like a big duck. This is not a familiar sight at the Science Center.

I moved on to Harvard Yard, where the trees were finally beginning to put out tentative buds. The trees must have known this was risky. One hard frost, a week's unusual chill, could kill off the tender green shoots and leave the trees to struggle through a difficult summer. I walked up to one tree and put my hands against its bark, congratulating it on its courage, trying to draw on its strength. The tree was warm under my hands. I swear I felt it communicating back to me, with its own brand of comfort and compassion. Even with an IQ of 3, it had things to teach me. I had come to believe that without any sense of false modesty.

After walking around in this contemplative daze for half the morning, I went back to William James Hall and took the elevator to the Sociology floor. I had missed the gender seminar. I was also becoming increasingly certain that I would not be able to put aside the tempest in my mind long enough to complete the research for my thirty-page term paper. I dimly remembered that five years, one year, ten months ago, failing to turn in a paper on time would have been unthinkable to me, unforgivable. Now it seemed trivial. I decided to explain my situation to one of the seminar's instructors and ask her for an incomplete on my transcript. This would buy me until two months after Adam's birth in which to research and write my paper.

The course instructor, an assistant professor, was in her office surrounded by a colorful chaos of books, papers, and greeting cards left over from the holidays. I waited outside in the hall while she finished a phone call. Given a few minutes to float free, my mind zipped right back to the strange new structure of my reality the way your tongue goes to a new filling, exploring its shape and dimension. Maybe Plato was right, I thought. Maybe we really do live in a dark place, a shadow world, a cave. The things I'd thought to be improbable, nonexistent, ghostly, insubstantial—all of these were quite possibly more real than the physical things I could see with my physical eyes.

I suddenly developed a craving to go back and read Plato—to read the work of any mystic, past or present. This seemed much more pressing than the reading for my gender seminar. It increased the electrical feeling that seemed to have become my constant companion. The initial jolt that had run through me the night before, when John said the name Adam, had never quite faded. It stayed with me all that night, through my wandering morning, and into my meeting with the seminar instructor. It waxed and waned, at times a barely perceptible tingle, at others a rush of energy so strong it made my heart thump like a kettledrum. I walked into the office still prickling with it.

It took me less than five minutes to state my case. I confessed that I hadn't been able to focus on the course content, that my attendance had been somewhat spotty, and that I couldn't concentrate long enough to write a check, let alone a term paper. The assistant professor didn't take much convincing. She already knew the basic facts about my pregnancy, my ill health, and the baby's Down syndrome.

"So," I said after I'd laid it all out, "would you be willing to give me an incomplete instead of failing me?"

"Sure," said the instructor. Then she stopped. She got a disconcerted look in her eyes, which appeared to be focused somewhere behind and above me. The electric feeling swelled until I shivered inside my maternity clothes.

"No," said the instructor slowly. "No, I'm not going to give you an incomplete. I'm going to give you an A."

"An A?"

She nodded.

"Surely you jest," I said. "I mean, I appreciate it, but . . ." I was going to say that I didn't deserve an A, which was true, but my voice trailed off. The professor didn't seem to be hearing me, not at all. She wasn't even looking at me. She was moving like a robot.

Now, just to assure the folks at Harvard that they don't need to track me down and revoke my Ph.D., I must tell you that I did in fact complete every bit of the work for that course. In fact, I have never been so motivated to write a term paper in my life. I finished it late, but I didn't have to go back and cope with the bureaucratic process of turning an incomplete into a letter grade. The most probable reason for this is that the instructor was a kind person. I happen to know that this is true (I also happen to know that after a semester or two she already hated Harvard). But since then, I have often seen people's native kindness spike upward just when I feel that strange electrical force surge in the air around me. The sensation has become a cue to me that something like this is about to happen.

I like to think that this means there are angels at work. As to the nature and identity of the angels, I'll accept as many interpretations as you like. Maybe the instructor for that gender seminar was, herself, an angel. Maybe there were invisible angels in the room, pushing on her psyche, nudging her toward magnanimity. Maybe they were my own, court-appointed guardian angels. Maybe Adam was the angel, as the Magna psychic said. Or maybe the answer is (D) All of the above.

For now, it's enough for me to think that angels, or for that matter any forms of goodness, function like water; they run into any opening they are given. There may be some people who are born open, who soak up goodness like sponges and leave traces of it on everything they touch. But even when an ordinary person (like me), or a bad person (like, say, Hitler), has a moment of openness, a moment of compassion, goodness rushes in to fill that space, to make us capable of receiving grace and transmitting it. Mother Teresa called this being "a pencil in the hand of God." There have been times when I have felt this way, as though I were being used as an instrument of goodness.

These moments are rare for me, and mostly accidental. I think that they are much more frequent for Adam.

The psychic from Magna may be right; Adam may be a kind of angel. But I don't think he's the only kind. Since that night on the sofa with John, I have come to believe that there are infinite passageways out of the shadows, infinite vehicles to transport us into the light. One of my favorite authors, Anne Lamott, quotes Rumi, a Persian mystic. As he wrote:

> *God's joy moves from unmarked box to unmarked box,*
> *from cell to cell. As rainwater, down into flowerbed.*
> *As roses, up from ground.*
> *Now it looks like a plate of rice and fish,*
> *now a cliff covered with vines,*
> *now a horse being saddled.*
> *It hides within these,*
> *till one day it cracks them open.*

With only a few weeks left until Adam's birth, I was well and truly cracked.

29

A friend of mine, who comes from a very religious home and has a daughter with Down syndrome, once told me that her mother blamed her for not miraculously transforming her little girl into a "normal" child. The logic was that if only my friend had enough faith, God would somehow suck the extra twenty-first chromosome out of every cell in the kid's body. My friend tried, but all the faith she could muster proved insufficient. She felt very guilty about that. It's amazing what can make people feel guilty.

If the theory espoused by my friend's mother is correct, and parents really can transform their children just by the power of belief, then the eighth month of my pregnancy must have been mighty strange for Adam. He must have spent his days morphing rapidly back and forth, like a character on Saturday morning cartoons; now the Barefoot Boy with Cheeks of Tan, now the Hunchback of Notre Dame. Most of the time I accepted the results of the amniocentesis: Adam has Down syndrome, and there was nothing I could do to fix it. But often, when the fear and sadness became unbearable, I would go back in my mind to all the miracles that had recently occurred around me and pray for just one more—a doozy. I created elaborate fantasies in which the delivering obstetrician hauled Adam out and shouted, "Oh my God, we made a terrible mistake—this baby is absolutely normal! In fact, he seems much stronger and healthier than any other baby I've ever delivered! I think he will win a Heisman Trophy and a Nobel Prize!"

It was especially important—and difficult—for me to find ways of coping when John was out of town. He took off for Singapore again in late April, leaving Sibyl to provide me with food and company. Sibyl and I had grown pretty darn close by then, what with all the dark hours during which I anticipated everything bad that could ever happen to Adam in his entire life, and she kept telling me that somehow things were going to be all right. Her tolerance for this kind of thing still astounds me.

Sibyl got a much-needed respite when I took Katie to my eldest sister's house in Florida for spring break. Like everyone else in my family, Christina walks around in a fairly brittle shell, communicating mainly in sarcasm, puns, and analytical theories. Underneath that, though, is enormous warmth, and a capacity for empathy so strong that when my sister sees people in pain, she seems to suffer more than they do. That spring she joked and debated with me as usual, but I could see how raw she was under the surface. We didn't talk much about the baby, mostly because I knew that if I started to cry, my sister might just not be able to go on living. She was thinking about Adam, though. One day she casually tossed me an article she had ripped out of a magazine. It was about a computer-enhanced way to help nonverbal disabled people communicate. According to the article, one teenager with Down syndrome, who had never spoken intelligibly, learned how to type out his thoughts using this system. The magazine quoted one of his first sentences, which was, "I hear God's finest whisper." I carried the article back to the guest bedroom to read it. Then I took a shower, so that I could stand under the water and cry for a while without spoiling anybody's day.

On Easter morning, Christina swamped Katie with more presents than she'd received at Christmas. Katie, needless to say, was thrilled. It was better than Christmas not only in terms of her total gift haul but also because she wasn't expecting it. She didn't even know the word *Easter*— she kept showing me everything she'd gotten from the Mister Bunny. What little I had taught her about the holiday was mainly concerned with the connection between eggs and rabbits and ancient Celtic fertility rites. For much of my life, the story of the Resurrection figured primarily as the basis for a tasteless joke in which Christ comes forth from the tomb, sees his shadow, and goes back in for six more weeks of winter.

Given my recent experiences and my new philosophy of life, I sat around my sister's house playing Prod with Adam and wondered if the story of Christ's resurrection could be literally true. I thought the same thing about the stories of the Buddha and Mohammed (my beliefs have never been exclusionary enough to make me a really good Christian). One thing that was powerfully attractive about the Greatest Story Ever Told, however, was the link between Jesus and miraculous healing. Like my friend's mother, I toyed with the idea that Adam might be "cured" through divine intervention. I actually spent a fair amount of time wondering how God would choose which of Adam's three twenty-first chromosomes would have to go. I figured that any combination of two, minus the third, would result in a slightly different person. This is how one begins to think after eight months of nausea and several weeks of grieving.

I was so ill and disassociated during that trip to Christina's house that I kept breaking things. I backed my sister's car out of her garage without opening the door first, causing damage to both the vehicle and the garage door. I fell asleep and let Katie wander around unsupervised, until I was awakened by the sound of something valuable shattering on the floor in the next room. I caused hundreds of dollars' worth of damage during my brief stay in Florida. My sister let me pay for some of it. By the time I left to return to Cambridge, I had added guilt to my long list of onerous emotions. I sincerely regretted that my family of origin hadn't just knocked me over the head and raised a good pig.

While Katie and I were destroying property in Florida, John was working flat-out to finish the consulting project in Singapore. The rest of the consultants on his team, who had been living in Asia during the entire project, were jubilant about their impending return to the United States. There were several of them, all Ivy League–educated, all young, all ambitious. Very ambitious. These people made Macbeth look like a monk. Ambition was what kept the junior consultants at the office virtually around the clock as the Singapore project neared completion. It catalyzed many watercooler conversations about the internal politics at headquarters, about what the members of the Asia team could expect when they returned to Boston, how they could get in with the right people at the top and, eventually, climb to the top themselves. The none-too-subtle competition among the individuals on the team picked up more speed and heft as the time to go home approached. As one consultant told John, during another interminable workday, "These are great guys. Good team players, yada yada. But if you ever shower next to one of them at the gym, don't bend over to pick up the soap."

The more intensely the team focused on their ambitions, the less John fit in. For one thing, he was constantly preoccupied with thoughts about me, Katie, and the new baby. None of his co-workers, not even the few married ones, ever talked about family members. Doing so would give too much ground to the next Young Turk in line, the one who might not be diverting his attention to domestic concerns. You had to cover your back.

Then there was the whole issue of the voices John had heard, of the dreamlike experience in the Tokyo shrine, of all the strange things I had told him were happening to me. Sometimes, when he allowed himself to think about these things, John would completely lose his focus on his work, until his colleagues—excuse me, his competitors—would snap their fingers or wave their hands in front of him, trying to wake him from his trance.

No matter how hard he tried to concentrate, things like this kept happening. He seemed to be standing outside some invisible wall that enclosed his fellows, keeping them in a sphere of concern and aspiration to which John was now a stranger. He knew he had been just like the other guys once, but he couldn't even remember what that had felt like—actually, he didn't think it had *felt* like anything at all. Feeling was not high on the list of priorities for a star executive. Now John was feeling, feeling acutely, and although most of what he felt was painful, he couldn't imagine trading it in for the anesthetized, driven, merciless focus on success that had once been his everyday condition. He remembered what Andrew Carnegie had once said: "Show me a contented man, and I'll show you a failure." This used to make sense to John. Now it seemed to beg the question of what a *successful* man must be.

Needless to say, John kept these thoughts to himself. If he'd confided in any of his peers, they could have ripped him apart. They were fully invested in the rat race, fighting desperately for the best spot in the cage—say, the one by the water spigot. John himself had fought with all his strength for such a spot. Now, events seemed to have ejected him from the cage, and instead of a bleak wasteland, he found himself in a world rich with possibility. To trade that for even the best shot at the spigot seemed absurdly undesirable.

⌐ A few days before John was scheduled to leave the Singapore office for the last time, he went to lunch with a rather large rat, an executive I'll call Carver. Although Carver was not a member of John's company, he was no stranger to consulting. John had met him on an assignment and considered him something of a mentor. Carver, being a Texan of adventurous ilk, had asked John to take him to a hawker center for lunch. John was more than happy to comply. Food hawkers, who used to stroll carts around the streets of Singapore, sell the best quick eating from Indian, Chinese, Malaysian, and some Western cultures. They are confined to small areas now, for sanitation and convenience. The air in these places is so fragrant it can almost make you swoon.

John and Carver sat down by a stand selling kway teow, which is a truly celestial concoction of rice noodles, beef, and garlic sauce. Once the food arrived and John's companion had downed a liter of beer, Carver began giving his usual career advice.

"Seems to me you've lost your focus," said the older man, looking at John with one eyebrow lowered.

"Maybe." John sighed. "It's been a tough year, you know, with . . . with this new baby coming and everything." John hadn't told Carver about the Down syndrome. He hadn't told anybody at work.

"Well, that right there proves my point," said Carver. "You should be letting Martha worry about the baby. You're a man, son! That's not where your focus should be."

John shrugged and shoveled in a little kway teow with his chopsticks.

The dish is spicy enough to sear your lips right off, but due to another head cold, John could barely taste it.

"What you want to do is get back to Boston, get in on another key project, and push like hell all the way from there to a senior-level consulting position. You've got to stay hungry."

"Uh-huh," said John wearily.

"I'm not fooling with you here," said Carver intently. "You've got to want it more than the next guy. That's the only thing that sorts out the men and the boys at this level."

John found his attention wandering. He looked around him. The hawker center was under a big awning, like a circus tent. Beneath the awning swarmed a kaleidoscope of color, scent, and sound. Half-naked Chinese chefs were sweating over woks on open fires; boys with huge black eyes and colorful sarongs served biryani to Indian customers; Islamic Malaysian women, their heads covered by scarves, fed exotic fruits into juicers and sold the nectar in little plastic bags.

"You know I'm right," said Carver.

"Uh-huh," said John again. He was fuzzily aware that his mentor was continuing the lecture on How to Succeed in Business, but he didn't really care.

John was thinking about me. He was thinking about the time we'd spent in Singapore the year after we were married. We were poor as dirt, so poor we carried everything we owned in two book bags. For fourteen months neither of us owned a pair of leather shoes—the ten-cent rubber thongs that the hawkers wore seemed to work just fine in that climate. We used to spend hours on the second story of the double-decker buses, riding along with no particular destination but a lot of curiosity. That, it seemed to John, had been a better way to spend a year of his life than fighting for a space by the water spigot.

  Half a world away, in our cold Cambridge apartment, I was dreaming of the rain forest. Instead of subway cars and sirens, the deafening rasp of cicadas buzzed in my ears. I could smell all the spices of Southeast Asia. I was eating kway teow. This was strange, because I hadn't been able to eat anything like that for months now.

Slowly, I became aware of a squeezing sensation in my middle. It was barely perceptible at first but quickly grew stronger, until it began to seriously impair my enjoyment of the kway teow. I looked down, annoyed, and almost choked with fear. There was a boa constrictor wrapped around me. It was huge. It clearly planned to keep squeezing until one of us gave up the ghost.

I woke up struggling for air, as though I'd just spent several minutes underwater. The Singaporean scene from my dream disappeared, but the squeezing sensation continued. I felt as though someone very large had decided to wring me out like a wet towel.

The contraction that woke me up that night, five weeks before my due date, wasn't strong enough to make me panic. I was sure it didn't mean anything. It wasn't time yet. The typical human pregnancy lasts forty weeks. A fetus born before the thirty-seventh week is considered premature. Adam was thirty-five weeks along, more than just a smidgen too young for life in the great outdoors. Many children with Down syndrome are born prematurely, and it does not help their chances for survival or normal functioning.

I told myself to calm down. It was only a Braxton Hicks contraction, I thought. A Braxton Hicks contraction is a sort of practice tightening of the uterus that occurs during the last weeks of pregnancy. These contractions are similar to actual labor but much less intense. They are called Braxton Hicks because they were "discovered" by a physician named, yes, Braxton Hicks. (What this actually means is that in the nineteenth century a man finally thought to attach his name to something that approximately 50 percent of the human race had been experiencing since the beginning of time. And you men wonder why we get so testy when we're pregnant.) I got up and took a Tums, which, along with chocolate and steak, had come to constitute its own food group in my prenatal diet. Then I lay down again and tried to sleep.

The second contraction came on very slowly. I told myself it was nothing but my imagination, until I felt Adam try to move and realized that my uterus had clenched around him like a fist. Don't panic, I thought. Mr. Braxton Hicks wouldn't want you to panic.

Twenty-five minutes after the second contraction, I had a third. Not close enough to mean anything. I lay down again, closed my eyes, rolled around on the stress mat for a while, and actually wished I could get back into my dream about the boa constrictor. It hadn't been all bad. At least I could eat spicy food in the dream—and now that I thought about it, John had been there. My eyes teared up when I thought about that. I missed him so much.

Poof.

I looked around the hawker center, at the blue-and-white-striped awning overhead and the skinny stray cats underfoot. It was very humid, as Singapore always is. Carver was waxing eloquent across the splattered tabletop, and the smell of spices wafted sumptuously through the crowd.

This time, for the first time, I was not simply dazzled by the experience of the Seeing Thing. I believed that it was real.

So I asked John to come home.

"Listen, honey," I whispered to the cold Cambridge night. "I need you. Please."

I think I expected the Seeing Thing to grow stronger then, like reception improving on a TV when you move the rabbit ears. Instead, the vision of the Singapore food court was suddenly gone, and I was left in the cold, dark apartment feeling like a fool. A fourth contraction hit, twenty minutes after the third.

⮂ "Play your cards right, and keep them close to your vest," Carver told John. "Very close."

They had finished eating and were polishing off the last of their drinks. John had been feigning attentiveness, throwing out the occasional "Uh-huh," and noticing, for the first time, that Carver didn't really care whether you listened to him or not, as long as he got to talk. John couldn't stop thinking about me, wishing I were the one sitting across from him. He began to miss me terribly. He closed his eyes and reminded himself that he'd be home in just three days. It seemed too long to wait.

"Hey!" Carver shouted to an Indian boy. "You there! Give us another beer!"

The boy came over to the table. He looked about ten, very slender, with deep brown skin and hair so black it shone blue. He said something to Carver in Tamil.

"I said *another beer*," Carver repeated, drawing out the words. "No speaky English?"

The boy looked confused, then broke into a shy smile. "English," he repeated.

"Good," said Carver. "Can you say *beer*?" He held up an empty bottle and swung it back and forth in front of the boy's face.

The boy brightened, nodding. "Beer," he repeated.

"That's right." Carver nodded approvingly. "Now, can you say, *I am stupid? I am ignorant? I have no class?*" He bellowed with laughter as the boy gave him a perplexed frown and went back to his stall to get the beer.

"Retards," Carver muttered to John. "In case they haven't noticed, English is their national language."

"Shut up," said John.

Carver froze, staring. He was almost as shocked as John was.

"I mean—listen, I'm sorry, Carver," John stammered, although come to think of it, he wasn't sorry at all. "My nerves are a little on edge," he concluded weakly. That was true. He was extremely edgy, because the voice that had just come out of his mouth, the one that told his mentor to shut up, seemed to have come *through* him, without being under his control.

"Whatever," said Carver archly, holding up his hands, palm forward. "Whatever. Didn't mean to offend."

John rubbed a hand across his brow. It was damp. "Listen," he said, "I've got to go home."

Carver looked at him with concern. "Okay, son," he said. "You don't look too well. I'll go back to the hotel with you."

"No." John shook his head. "I mean *home*. I've got to get home." This, too, seemed to come through his vocal cords almost before he knew what he was going to say. As he paid the check and hurried to hail a taxi, John knew that he'd be on a plane that afternoon.

Back at his hotel, while he threw his belongings into the hanging bag he always carried, he thought over the few remaining tasks necessary to complete his portion of the consulting project. As he recalled each detail of the work, he instantly saw a way that it could be performed by phone, fax, or mail. There was nothing that really required him to stay in Singapore. This was fortunate, because John's body appeared to have decided to leave the country with or without his consent. He heaved the strap of his hanging bag onto his shoulder and sprinted for the exit as if he'd heard a starter's gun.

It took him less than fifteen minutes to check out, but when he left the hotel, he saw that the line for a taxi was thirty people long. A bellboy was whistling cabs over, one by one, at a leisurely pace.

John carried his hanging bag up to the bellboy. "I need a taxi right now," he said. "It's an emergency." He still had that bizarre, out-of-control sensation. He felt as though he were not the one who had ordered the cab. If I'd been there, I could have told him it was only the puppeteers.

"Sorry, sir," said the bellboy. "Queue up, please."

"No." John was almost pleading. "I've got to get home *now*. Please."

The man shook his head. "Sorry, sir. Queue up, please." He was a small man, short and very slender. He was wearing a uniform that looked like a cross between a suit of armor and a Victorian party dress. The spike of his helmet barely came up to John's nose.

"I'll give you twenty dollars," said John. The bellboy's eyes flickered, first at John, then at the people waiting behind him. The other customers were all watching. The man shook his head.

John didn't know what to do, especially since he didn't understand why he was doing it. He forced himself to think. He had been through thousands of hours of instruction at Harvard, had read millions of words and written thousands more, all to learn how to do business in Asia. He knew everything there was to know about bridging the cultural divide with empathy and sensitivity. He should be able to come up with a plan, he thought, but nothing came to his mind. Instead, John watched, transfixed, as his hands leapt out of their own accord and grabbed the bellboy's collar ruffle.

"Get me a taxi, right now," John said, "or I'll kill you."

The crowd gasped in horror. The bellboy gasped in horror. John gasped in horror. He barely had time to begin apologizing before the bellboy blew a piercing blast on his whistle, opened the door of the next cab in line, and fairly shoved John into it. He was halfway to Changi Airport before the strange sensation in his hands and throat subsided, and his body reverted to his control.

Later, when John told me about how his body had driven off without him, had taken matters literally into its own hands, I knew just how he'd felt. Because that's exactly what it feels like when you're having a baby.

30

❧ John had a lot of trouble getting home. It just so happened that the very day he bolted from Singapore was the beginning of a Japanese holiday period known as Golden Week. This one week contains no fewer than three important holidays, all of which mandate travel to one's place of birth. The Japanese travelers during this one week clog up the entire Asian air travel industry. Imagine throwing Thanksgiving Day in between Christmas and New Year's, and you'll have some idea of the logistical problems one might encounter traveling through Asia during Golden Week. The Singapore airport was so packed that the lines extended through the outer doors. The building teemed with Japanese expatriates heading home for the week, as well as the usual Chinese tourists going back to the mainland, carrying live chickens and ducks in their luggage.

John fought his way to the business-class line at the Singapore Airlines counter. He waited in it for over an hour, and as he drew closer to the counter he heard several people ask to buy tickets without reservations. Not one of these people was successful. By the time John reached the counter, his prospects of getting a ticket back to the United States, which would necessitate going through other parts of Asia, were looking mighty dim.

"Is there any way I can get to the USA?" he asked.

"No, sir, I'm sorry," said the attendant. "Not until next week. All flights are completely booked."

John nodded dejectedly. "Could you check?" he said, without any real hope.

The attendant shrugged. "Well, all right, sir, but—oh, hold on! Jolly good!"

John liked the sound of that, even though it was odd to hear it spoken by an Asian. (Singaporean English is chock-full of British idioms.)

"I just had a cancellation," said the attendant. "An economy-class ticket. It goes right through from Singapore to New York City. Would you like it?"

Well, thought John, there you go again.

John still thinks God was behind that cancellation, that it was arranged specifically to get him back to Boston. He has always wondered, though, why God couldn't get him a better seat. He arrived in New England twenty-three hours later, having sat in the very back row of several flights, in a middle seat, between two men who smoked copiously and talked to each other constantly but would not give up their window and aisle seats to sit side by side. He had to stop in Bahrain, where he hoped the two men would deboard, but they got off the plane only long enough to buy more cigarettes.

⌐ Meanwhile, back at the ranch, I continued to have strong contractions every twenty minutes or so for a whole day. I'd been to University Health Services, where the obstetrician on call said that my cervix wasn't dilated and that I should go home and rest. Sibyl and Deirdre had, of course, called every hour or so and come by when they could, in case things progressed any further. When night fell and the contractions were still twenty minutes apart, I phoned them both and told them to go to bed. I promised I would call if anything changed.

Nothing did. After Katie fell asleep, I found myself once again on the stress mat, dozing fitfully for twenty minutes at a time. Saying that I was worn out would be like saying that the World Trade Center is a split level with a decent view. I was *trashed*. I had started praying, had actually gotten quite used to it, but that night I didn't know what to pray for. I lay on the stress mat and felt a terrible struggle going on inside me. One part of me wanted desperately to end this torturous pregnancy *now*, no matter what. Another part insistently reminded me that I had to keep Adam in the oven until he was well done, or at least medium rare.

I was not my best self when John came in at 3:00 A.M. He looked as bad as I felt. He had two and a half days of beard stubble on his chin, and his eyes were so bloodshot from cigarette smoke that he looked like one of the undead from a bad B movie.

I didn't care. When I heard John's key click in the door of our apartment, all the tension I had been holding back came bursting out of me. I was safe again, safe enough to fall apart, and that is what I did. As soon as John put his arms around me, in the doorway of the bedroom, I began to sob like a drunk at her mother's funeral.

"I'm so scared, John," I told him when I could speak through my sobs. "I don't know what's going to happen and I'm so *tired* and I want to get it over with but I don't want to make it worse and I feel so awful and I don't know if I can handle having a baby like this and what if he's really sick or has to have surgery or life support or what if he dies or—"

"Calm down," John kept saying. "Are you still having contractions?"

"Yes," I said. "But it's too soon. If he's premature he'll be even more messed up."

"He's not going to be premature," John said, "and he's not going to be messed up. Remember all the things that have happened to you? To us?"

I nodded.

"I believe he could be healed," said John. "I do."

"He's not sick, really." I wiped my face with the sleeve of my bathrobe. "Doesn't need healing, exactly."

"Well, maybe *fixed* is a better word," John said.

I looked into his red, sunken eyes. "You really believe that could happen?"

He nodded, his eyes very tired but steady. "Look at everything else that's going on," he said. He thought for a minute, and then said, "You were with me in Singapore, weren't you?"

I had almost stopped crying. I nodded. "At the hawker center. You had kway teow."

John gave a low, astonished chuckle. "Damn," he said. "Even though I knew it worked, it's incredible. Isn't it incredible?"

I finally smiled, the first smile I'd managed in two days. "Yeah," I said. "I guess it is."

"So." John gave me his own quick grin. "Why not believe that other incredible things can happen? Good things?"

I couldn't answer him. Another contraction was under way, and I was trying hard to relax and breathe through it. "I just wish I were sure," I whispered, once the pain had passed. "I just want to *know*. All those little miracles are nice, but they're not enough."

John slid me from his lap to the stress mat as though he were putting Katie to bed. "Martha, Martha." He sighed. "What am I gonna do with you? You know, there are millions of people in this world who would give anything just to experience some of the things that have happened to you over the past little while."

I nodded, too tired to talk.

"Most people go through their whole lives," John went on, "and never have one miracle happen to them. You've had dozens and dozens, and you still want more! It's like God gives you a brownie, I mean a really *good* brownie, but you can't be content with it. You want the whole *pan* of brownies. Nobody gets that."

"Maybe so," I said. "Maybe so. But I still want it."

John shook his head, laughing. "You are a case, Martha Beck," he said. "You are a genuine case." He arranged a pillow under my head.

"Get some sleep now," he said.

I lay there for ten minutes or so, waiting for him to come to bed with me. He didn't. I could hear him puttering around the apartment, first in the kitchen, then in the bathroom. I was almost asleep when another contraction gripped me and my body flooded with adrenaline. When it was over I got up and waddled down the hall.

"John?" I said. "Are you coming to bed?"

"No," he answered. "Not now." He was still in the bathroom. He had dumped out the contents of the laundry hamper on the floor and was sorting the clothes by color.

"Aren't you tired?" I said, poking my head through the door. "You look awfully tired. You look like a sick terrorist."

John flashed his weary smile again. "I am tired," he said, "but it's midday in Singapore. I couldn't fall asleep right now if I tried. Thought I'd get the laundry done instead."

I didn't bother to contradict him, but I knew what he was really doing. He was comforting himself with work, as he had always done. I figured this was a better addiction than drugs or alcohol, so I didn't ask him to come to bed again. I watched while John sorted the dark clothes into a pile and pushed them into an empty pillowcase. He slung the pillowcase full of clothes onto his back and told me he'd be back from the laundry room in a few minutes. I was reluctant to let him go even that long. When the apartment door closed behind him, I finally accepted that no matter who was around me, no matter how helpful and loving people tried to be, I was still going to end up facing my fears alone.

I walked into the living room and sat down on the floor, looking out over Harvard Square. I sat in the position the Japanese call *seiza*, with my rear end resting on my feet. It is a respectful posture, almost like kneeling. I clasped my hands over my enormous belly and tried to talk to God.

"Listen," I said. "I'm sorry the brownies you've given me aren't enough. I'm sorry I'm so weak. But I can't do this anymore."

Another contraction hit, and I had to stop talking. When it passed, I felt so exhausted that I almost fell over sideways.

"I'm sorry," I gasped again, "but I *can't*. It's too much for me. Please. Please."

⟿ What I remember most about that moment was a sense of letting go. For the first time, I prayed without trying to control whatever the answer might be. I was just too tired to hang on, to control anything. It was almost like getting out of the driver's seat of a car and handing someone else the keys: "Hey, I'm sozzled. In no shape to get behind the wheel. Maybe you should drive." I had been drunk for years, on the illusions I had thought meant happiness. I had drunk myself into oblivion on prestige and intellect and praise. I was in no shape to be driving my own life.

At the moment when I stopped fighting for control of my little universe, I noticed something that had been there all along, except that I hadn't seen it. It was slightly to the left of me, maybe eighteen inches off the floor. It was a person—or rather, a person's feet. That was all I saw— a pair of bare feet, standing in the air, with the hem of a robe falling around the ankles.

I didn't even bother to look up at the person's body or face. Some of the few people I told about this experience asked me why not. All I can say is that when you are reunited with the love of your life, you don't hold yourself at arm's length. This being wasn't unfamiliar to me at all. I wasn't surprised or stunned or frightened. I felt that the natural order of the universe had been restored, not disturbed, and I was immensely, over-whelmingly relieved. And so I simply leaned forward, letting my fore-head rest against those suspended feet, and began to cry like a child who had been found after being lost in a storm.

"I've waited so long," I sobbed. "I've waited so long."

I don't remember the slightest feeling of surprise. The situation didn't seem strange to me at all. I didn't want to stare, or run, or even wonder. In fact, what I would once have called my "normal" life—a life in which there seemed to be no spiritual beings around me—was the state of being that seemed bizarre to me now. It was absolutely clear, as clear as reality becomes when you waken from a dream, that I had been waiting all my life to be with this person again.

What amazed me more than the physical presence in the room was the love that came with it. I felt as though I were caught in a glowing tidal wave of love, a love so strong that all the pain on earth couldn't even begin to put a dent in it. I have sometimes wondered why I didn't feel cheated at having spent so many terrible days on earth before I found that love again. But once I was back within it, all the frustration and lone-liness I had ever suffered seemed completely inconsequential.

I was still crying, my forehead resting against those feet, when I felt two strong hands reach under my arms and pull me gently upward. I had the impression that I was being lifted out of my body, which was still kneeling on the floor. I felt connected to it, in a distant way, but not inside it. It was only, after all, a woman of earth, wrapped around a child of earth. I, the part of me that constitutes my identity, was lifted away from it, into an embrace so sweet that for years and years it never for a single second left my mind. Still today, when I hear a song on the radio about finding the ultimate love, the perfect love, the love one cannot live without, I think about that being who picked me up and held me like a baby, on that chilly spring night near Harvard Square.

I don't know how long it lasted; maybe thirty seconds, maybe ten minutes. Not more than that. Whatever it was, my entire existence still hinges on that brief encounter. It is the center point for me, the single event that divides my life into Before and After.

I don't know how unusual it is to experience this kind of thing. It's not something you want to run out and recount to the neighbors over pound cake and tea. If it is rare, I would guess that its rarity has to do with the immense difficulty it brings into your life. I know this sounds strange. I always used to think that if I just *knew* there was Someone Out There, if I had some evidence of a Higher Power that I could trust completely, life would be a bowl of cherries. Nope. If you have ever experienced something like this, you know that it doesn't automatically make the rest of your experience easy to tolerate. On the contrary, after tasting that kind of love, that kind of belonging, it is almost unbearable to feel separated from it again.

In the months and years after this experience I would practice every form of religious and mystical discipline that I thought might have the slightest chance of bringing me back into the presence of that overwhelming love. A lot of mystics fast; I would go days without eating. Others meditate; I spent hours and hours—at night, when the kids and John were asleep—clearing my mind and waiting for the Being to return. I kept every rule of every religion I knew anything about. I was kosher and halal and vegetarian. I didn't smoke, drink, or swear. I gave money to the poor. I tried to be kind to everyone and everything, to the point of groveling, although my motives were purely selfish.

Most of all, though, I fell in love with the thought of death. I was in no way suicidal, but I believed that death was the one sure passage back into the presence of that love, and I could hardly wait. A few years later,

I confided this whole experience to a woman who had "died" of a heart attack. She'd gone through the whole near-death thing, with the tunnel and the light and so on. Given a choice whether to live or die, this woman decided on a compromise: she'd come back to life just long enough to give her children a few instructions, then die again. "I'll be right back," she assured the Being of Light. When she came to, in her body of clay, she was outraged to find that a crew of paramedics had shocked her heart back into its regular pattern. It took her a long time to get over the intense disappointment of living. She told me she takes great comfort from knowing she gets to die again.

For a full three years after God gave me a whole pan of brownies, the thing I wanted most in the world was to die. I was half crazy with longing for it. I guess I got so obsessive that the Powers That Be concluded I needed something to knock me back on track, like the Skipper whacking Gilligan on the head to correct the amnesia caused by a previous whack on the head.

So I got another pan of brownies.

At the time, Adam was three and a half, and my health was lousy. What with my still undiagnosed autoimmune disease and all the fasting and the death wish and so forth, my body kept breaking down and requiring surgery for one thing or another. During one of these operations, I suddenly found myself alert and aware and gazing at a brilliant white light that had appeared directly above my head. The light was shaped like a sphere, not a person, but there was no doubt in my mind that it was the same being who had held and comforted me that night in my apartment. I started to cry from pure joy, alarming the surgeons, who knew I was still under general anesthesia. The anesthesiologist would have sedated me even further, except that the light told him not to, assuring him that I was crying because I was happy. (That doctor came and talked to me after the surgery, to ask me what in the world had been going on, and later wrote to me about the experience.)

While the surgery proceeded, the Being of Light gently explained to me that I was barking up all the wrong trees. I would not find my way back home by fasting, it told me, or by meditating, following endless lists of rules, or even dying. All those things might help, given the right conditions, but not unless I was willing to do something much more difficult.

The light didn't use words—I simply knew what it wanted to tell me—and so it's hard for me to explain in words what it communicated. I tried to tell John, after the surgery, and he assumed I was babbling through a drugged haze, which was true. However, there was a concrete message that remained even after the drugs had left my system, and this is—sort of—what it said. It said that the way back to my real environment, the place where my soul was meant to exist, doesn't lie through any set of codes I will ever find outside of myself. I have to look inward. I have to jettison every sorrow, every terror, every misconception, every lie that stands between my conscious mind and what I know in my heart to be true. Instead of clutching around me all the trappings of a "good" person, a "successful" person, or even a "righteous" person, I have to be exactly what I am, and take the horrible chance that I may be rejected for it. I can't get home by cloaking myself in the armor of any system, social, political, or religious. I have to strip off all that comforting armor and go on naked.

✑   Back in late April of 1988, I was so stunned by the flood of love that swept me off our living room floor that I couldn't yet begin to put words around it. By the time John came back in and rinsed the laundry soap off his hands, the living room was dark again and the sirens blared through the night beyond Harvard Yard. I was back in a world where death and taxes are the only sure things, where the fear of oblivion taints every moment of consciousness, where we struggle and struggle and struggle against entropy, knowing every second that we are losing the battle. I was back in the shadow world.

Sibyl would tell me later that she hadn't really worried about me until after that night. "You seemed to be going through a normal grieving process," she said, "and then, all of a sudden, you just *stopped.*"

It was true. I was completely dazed. Trying to integrate the immensity of that love into my mind and heart became my full-time occupation for months. When the being disappeared, leaving a residue of love on every surface in my apartment, my uterus was still contracting enthusiastically. But my fear, and the sense of pitched battle, were gone. I no longer worried about going into labor. I felt utterly trustful that things were under control, though no control of mine. I was willing to bet that between them, Adam and the Being of Love probably had some kind of plan. Whatever it was, I was in it for the duration.

31

↶ I hung on for another week, the contractions gradually speeding up. Obviously, I didn't sleep a lot during that week, but then, I didn't really want to. I wanted to sit around and think about what had happened to me the Night of the Magic Feet. The peace from that moment glowed in me for a long time, making me want to hush everything and focus on it the way you would listen to very soft, supernally beautiful music. People who knew me well started to wonder if I had gained access to some sort of recreational drug.

Even with the warmth and wonder to shore me up, the repetitive stress of those endless contractions slowly eroded my endurance. I had a distinct feeling that I was postponing Adam's birth deliberately, that if I decided to let go, he'd pop right out. I was determined to hang on to him until the thirty-seventh week of gestation. It wasn't the easiest thing I've ever done.

While I lay around, watching *Sesame Street* with Katie and trying to carry Adam to term, John was busy finalizing all his business at the consulting company. He had arranged a meeting on the seventh of May with the man who had hired him. John had decided to quit. I knew how much this hurt him, how deeply it felt like failure. I remembered how excited we had both been when he'd gotten the job, and how intent he'd been on proving himself. Nevertheless, we were both coming to accept the idea that our lives would be very different once Adam was born. We weren't sure exactly what it would be like, but we were sure that our burden as parents would be much heavier, and that John wouldn't have the kind of freedom he'd need to succeed in such a competitive industry. Ever since the night he'd spent in the Japanese shrine, John had known which way his choices would take him. But that wasn't the easiest thing *he'd* ever done, either.

John kissed me good-bye that morning, carried Katie out to the elevator, and took her over to Sibyl's house so that I could get some rest. When they were gone the apartment felt too empty, too silent, and too dirty. It had been a mess for months, but now the need to clean it took on a sudden urgency. I'd begun to experience the "nesting" urge that precedes labor. There have been only three times in my life—once for each child—when I actually wanted to clean the refrigerator. This was one of them, another sign that labor was proceeding ahead of schedule. I held myself back, hoping that if I refused to nest, my body might not eject Adam quite so soon. The refrigerator sat there, humming to itself, taunting me with the smudges on its shelves.

I knew I was supposed to stay in bed, but I felt as if I'd go completely mad if I didn't do something. I dressed myself and hit the streets of Cambridge, bent on one thing: shopping. I decided that it might curb the nesting urge if I at least purchased a few feathers.

John and I were never very conscientious about preparing nurseries for our children. We had an unspoken suspicion that Something Bad Might Happen, a feeling that it was bad luck to count chickens that were still in the egg. When Katie was born, we hadn't even bought a blanket to wrap around her on her way home from the hospital. She slept in a dresser drawer until we managed to find a crib, a week later. Of course, our trust in Adam's chances at survival were even lower. We still had Katie's old crib and plenty of used blankets, but we didn't have one single article of clothing for a boy baby. On the bright May morning when John set off to quit his job, I decided I'd remedy that.

I waddled the half mile to the Harvard Coop, stopping and trying to look casual when a contraction came on. Once I got there I went straight to the insignia section. Neither John nor I had ever worn anything with "Harvard" written on it. It seemed so pretentious. We hadn't ever put any Harvard insignia on Katie, either, even though the sweatshirts and baseball caps looked adorable in baby sizes. But with Adam, I would break the mold. I was going to put the word *Harvard* all over that little retarded boy. I figured that any statement this made, about either Adam or Harvard, would be apropos.

The nesting energy that got me over to the Coop was pretty much gone by the time I got home, with a tiny "Harvard" sweatsuit in tow. The walk seemed to take forever. When our apartment door finally closed behind me, I leaned back against it and slid all the way to the floor. Another contraction hit. It was intense enough to make me grit my teeth.

"Um, God?" I said. I always talked this way now, whenever I was alone. "Listen, I know it's still a week early, but I'd really—oof."

The squeezing sensation was getting fiercer, too fierce to allow conversation.

"I'd really like to end this," I said, when I could. Then I waited. I didn't know what to expect; a voice from heaven, a burning bush, a talking pigeon. I didn't care. All I wanted was some sort of permission.

"So, how about it?" I asked the Great Beyond.

Nothing.

Eventually I heaved my bulky self up and proceeded to Katie's bedroom—I guess you could call it the nursery. There still wasn't much furniture in it; just the crib, a chest of drawers, and an easy chair so battered that it had been left in the apartment by the previous tenants. I went to the chest of drawers and opened the bottom drawer, the one where I'd stored all Katie's outgrown clothes and baby blankets. I was going to put Adam's little "Harvard" sweatsuit underneath everything else, so that John wouldn't see it. Then, if the baby died, I could dispose of it on my own. No one would ever have to know.

I was pushing the clothes aside, digging for the very bottom of the drawer, when I heard the rustle of a plastic bag. I frowned, curious, and dug further. Underneath the blankets and T-shirts and sleep suits I found a small package. The bag bore the label of a Singaporean sporting goods store, one that sold Western products at near-black-market prices. Inside was a tiny pair of Reebok tennis shoes. They were exact replicas of the adult versions, hardly bigger than your thumb, as miniature and perfect as two matched hummingbirds. Shoes like that are common in the United States now, but I'd never seen anything like them. I took them out of their packaging and held them, one in each hand. They felt solid and surprisingly heavy, the way a sleeping baby does. I put them up to my face and realized I was crying. That was the first time since Adam's diagnosis that I realized how desperately I wanted him to live.

∽ Two miles away, John was having another of those bizarre conversations, the ones that never happen in real life, the ones where God descends directly out of the machine and fixes some difficult situation while the chorus chants its approval. Later, when John described it to me, I couldn't stop thinking about the strange look on my Sociology of Gender instructor's face the day she had insisted on giving me an A.

John's meeting that afternoon was with a man named Mark Fuller, one of the company's founders. Mark was not your typical business executive; he was a quixotic dreamer, thoughtful and innovative, a man who inhaled books and listened intently to everyone he ran across, from CEOs to tollbooth attendants. I had met him when I was noticeably pregnant with Katie, and he had immediately begun to describe to me his idea for an in-house day-care center at the consulting firm. This was the man who had hired John, and both of us respected him. One of the main reasons John regretted quitting was that he felt he was failing Mark.

After some initial pleasantries, John cut to the chase. "I came in today to resign," he said.

Mark stared at him. "What?"

"I think we'll probably be moving," said John. "Our baby is due in a month, and I think we should be around family. It would be best for my wife." He winced when he heard himself, remembering the way Carver had reacted to him in Singapore.

Mark still looked stunned. "I'm not sure I understand," he said. "You never mentioned this before."

"Yes. Uh, well . . ." John cleared his throat. "In the last few weeks we've . . . we've gotten more information."

Mark shook his head. "John, what are you talking about?"

There didn't seem to be any way out of it. John took a deep breath. "The baby has Down syndrome," he said.

Mark's eyes widened even more. "Oh, my God," he said. "Are you sure?"

John nodded glumly. "Amniocentesis," he said. "Hundred percent accuracy."

As John recalls it, Mark's own wife was pregnant at that time. That may have been why Mark became very pensive at this point in the conversation, falling silent and pacing back and forth, as he often did when presented with a problem.

"Are you finished with your dissertation?" he asked suddenly.

John felt lower than slug slime. "No," he said. Not "I'm very close," not "The research is locked away," not "Ninety-five percent." John was tired of giving everything a successful spin, especially now, when he thought the real odds of his completing his degree program were slim to none. He had to find steady work to support us all, and that didn't leave much time for academic research.

"How long would it take you to finish the dissertation," Mark asked, "assuming that you had nothing else to do?"

John thought for a minute. "Six months, give or take."

"Okay, okay," said Mark. "How about this: We'll pay you as a full-time employee for six months while you finish your dissertation."

John opened his mouth and then closed it again. "And?" he managed to stammer.

"And then we'll still have a relationship with you," said Mark. "Professionally."

He seemed very pleased with this idea. John thought it through carefully and could find in it virtually no financial "upside" for the company.

"I'm not sure I understand," he said at last.

"Your dissertation will do the company good," said Mark, although he did not specify exactly how. Nevertheless, he seemed to mean it. He was, after all, the only person John had ever met who would actually read a Ph.D. dissertation for pleasure.

"I don't know what to say," John stammered, half-expecting Mark to smile sweetly, yank out a magic wand, and tell him to click his heels together three times.

"How about yes?" said Mark.

"Okay," said John. "Okay, yes. Yes!"

Mark extended his hand. "Resignation denied." He beamed.

John reached forward with his own hand, feeling dizzy and surreal. It was as though he had come up too quickly from the depths of the ocean, from a place where intense pressure had been crushing in on him, to some mellow, bounteous Fantasy Island. For the first time in his life, John thought he might be about to faint.

That's how everything went when we were expecting Adam: bizarrely badly, or bizarrely well. Those puppeteers turned the whole damn world upside down. You might say that I am putting too much stock in the workings of spirit, in the will of God. You might say that John and I were simply discovering the goodwill that had lain, all along, in the hearts of some decent human beings. But you would be assuming that these two things are different, and that is an assumption I reject. I have been blessed with love both human and divine, and I believe that there is no essential difference between them. Any person who acts out of love is acting for God. There is no way to repay such acts, except perhaps to pass them on to others.

At about the time Mark Fuller was doing his Glinda the Good imitation, I was counting the days left until the magical thirty-seven-week gestation point. I didn't think I could hold the contractions at bay much longer. I put the little Harvard sweatsuit next to the tiny Reebok shoes in the bottom of Katie's hand-me-down drawer and crept into the bedroom to lie down.

"*Pack a bag,*" said a voice by my elbow.

All my hair stood on end. "What?"

"*Pack a bag.*"

I knew what it meant. I was supposed to get my things ready to take to the hospital.

I went to the closet and pulled out the bag I had used to heft all my belongings when John and I were newlyweds in Southeast Asia. Another contraction came on, hard. I put a robe into the bag, and a pair of slippers. Then I went to the bathroom and dug out an extra toothbrush, toothpaste, mouthwash, and a hairbrush.

"It's early," I said. "It's too early."

The voice said nothing. I went back into Katie's room and opened the bottom drawer again. I stood looking into it for some time, wondering if I would need any baby things, wondering if Adam would go directly into surgery as two out of five Down's babies do, wondering if yet another dreadful decision, or a series of them, lay ahead of me.

"What should I pack?" I asked. I didn't expect an answer, not really. But I got one.

"What do you think?"

"Would you cut that out?" I said fretfully. "Would you please, for once, just give me a direct answer?"

For just a moment, I had a flash of insight—or rather, outsight, where I could see myself from the perspective of the person I'd been a few short months before. I was standing in an empty room, not only talking to a disembodied voice but *arguing* with it. I'd left the typical definition of sanity so far behind that, although I saw the absurdity in this, it didn't even faze me.

The fact was that the voice was right. When I looked inside myself, I knew exactly how Adam's health was going to be. He would be fine. He wouldn't require surgery, wouldn't get sick very often, wouldn't even have the frequent ear infections we'd been warned are typical of kids with Down syndrome. Aside from his extra chromosome, he'd be a perfectly healthy little boy.

How did I know this? I just did. I have always liked Albert Einstein's comment that "people like us, who believe in physics, know that the distinction between past, present, and future is only a stubbornly persistent illusion." Every now and then I have had premonitions strong enough to convince me this is true in practice, not merely in theory.

I've experienced this kind of foreknowledge half a dozen times since Adam was born. It never happens when I try to force it. Instead, it pops up from nowhere when I meet a person who will later become important to me for one reason or another. It hits me like a brick when I visit a place I will later come to live. So far, this sense of knowing, which feels a lot like "remembering" something that is not past but future, has never been wrong. I don't think I'm unusual in having these premonitions. It's just that when I was expecting Adam I was lucky enough to be forced to notice them, and trust them. Of course, no matter how many times they prove correct, I am always afraid to trust them again. But in my more lucid moments I believe that if we pay attention, all of us occasionally bump into our own futures.

When John arrived home from his resignation excursion, staggering like a junkie with gratitude and relief, he found me poking around my premonitions like a child playing with a strange but fascinating animal. He rushed through the door, swept me up in his arms, and kissed me for a long time. He didn't even notice that he had to step over my packed bag, which was standing in the doorway.

"You know what, honey?" John said exuberantly. "The most incredible thing just happened! I think everything's going to be all right!"

I nodded. "I know it is."

"Listen." John grinned at me. "You're not going to believe this."

"Oh, I think I am. Whatever it is, I think I am."

"No, really," said John. "I have to tell you—"

"Sibyl and Charles are waiting for us in the parking lot," I interrupted. "Come on—you can tell me in the car."

"The car?" John looked puzzled.

"On the way to the hospital," I said. "This is it."

John's eyes and mouth opened wide. "But isn't it too soon for—"

"Don't worry," I said. "He'll be fine. Everything will be fine."

I said it with such conviction that John had no choice but to believe it.

32

↶ When John and I got to the parking lot, Sibyl, Charles, Mie, and Katie were waiting, the door of their car already open. We drove through a late-spring snow flurry to Brigham and Women's Hospital in Boston. Between my contractions, I smoothed Katie's hair and talked to her softly about what was happening. We'd discussed it all before, of course, but she listened with rapt attention, her blue eyes huge and solemn.

John had brought a little Japanese stopwatch with him in his coat pocket. Whenever a contraction came on, I'd tell him, "Now," and when it ebbed away, I'd say, "Over." John would check the stopwatch and let me know how long it had lasted, and how long the interim had been between it and the previous contraction. It sounded a little like Mission Control:

"Now."

"Over."

"One minute thirteen seconds."

"How long since the last one?"

"Ten fifty-three."

"Roger."

It was a half-hour drive. When it ended, I kissed Katie and told her that we'd call her on the phone later that night, while she stayed over at Mie's house. I thanked Sibyl and Charles, hoping they could sense the depth of my gratitude, since it was impossible to express in words. Then they pulled away, and John and I were on our own again.

I thought about how different this was from Katie's birth, which had felt like a party by comparison. I'd reacted to a shot of Demerol by seeing boats and horses in the delivery room. I don't remember it all that well, but John says I was a laugh riot. Once Katie was born, the party got even better. There was a small blizzard of happy phone calls and cards and flowers. John's Business School section took out a whole column in the *Harbus,* the HBS newspaper, to run a congratulatory ad that said

"The Section H class of 1986 welcomes Katherine Beck, class of 2010." The day I had Adam was as different from Katie's birthday as bungee jumping is from a high-risk rescue operation.

∽ I refused the offer of a wheelchair and paced back and forth in the hospital lobby while John filled out the entry forms. At one point, he came over and asked solicitously if it wouldn't be better for me to sit down. He pointed toward a small lobby, where a sign said PATIENT WAIT-ING. I told John that he knew I'd never been a patient person, especially not when waiting. If he could find an *im*patient waiting area, I'd be happy to patronize it. He grinned at me and went back to filling out forms. Within a few minutes, before he had finished, I'd run out of spunk. I sat down on one of the hideous orange vinyl chairs in the PA-TIENT WAITING lobby and curled up around my bulging torso. I didn't even argue much when a nurse rolled another wheelchair over and in-vited me to climb aboard.

The nurse walked beside us as John pushed the chair to the eleva-tor, then out onto the labor and delivery floor. She led us down a long, sterile-looking hallway to my assigned labor room. The hospital was busy that morning; most of the rooms along the hallway were already occu-pied. Nurses in white pantsuits and doctors in those blue pajamas with the little shower-cap hats bustled through the corridor. The maternity floor is generally the happiest place in any hospital. Even though the at-mosphere was eminently professional, people smiled more on that floor than any other. It made me feel simultaneously glad and wistful, cheered to be in a place where good things happen, scared that nothing good was going to happen for me and my family.

The room next to mine was particularly lively. Nurses rushed in and out like worker bees in a honeycomb, carrying various implements and linens. I couldn't see the expectant mother inside, but I could hear her. Everyone could hear her. This is what really bugs me about the labors you see on television; the tiny starlets who play expectant mothers gasp and moan when they're having their television babies, but on the whole they do it delicately. You rarely hear them bellowing like cows being led to the slaughter, which is how my next-door neighbor sounded. It was a truly awful noise, almost inhuman. John and I looked at each other in alarm.

"It's okay," our nurse said in a stage whisper. She jerked a thumb toward the room whence the bellowing-cow sounds were emanating, and added, "She's Hispanic." I nodded bleakly, too concerned by what lay ahead of me to challenge her political incorrectness.

As it turned out, I did my part to correct that nurse's impressions about Caucasian versus Hispanic reactions to the pain of childbirth. My stiff-lipped Nordic ancestors would no doubt have been appalled by the way I comported myself over the next few hours. I hadn't attended a Lamaze refresher course to prepare for Adam's birth—I didn't think I could handle going among so many "normal" pregnant women—but I remembered that before Katie was born, my Lamaze instructor had commented that the pain of labor is much worse if the mother is afraid. She was right. I wasn't frightened by the actual process of delivering Adam, but I was terrified of what might happen afterward. Between contractions I'd hold the fear at arm's length, but when the pain came on again, I'd just lose it. The next day I didn't recall much about my labor. I mentioned to John that I had a sore throat, but I couldn't figure out why. He just looked at me and said, "Duh."

At one point I remember a nurse (who was probably about to offer me a little Demerol, to take the edge off the contractions) coming into the room, parking herself next to the bed, and saying, "Don't think about the pain, dear. Just think about the baby. Think about that wonderful, beautiful, perfect little baby you're going to have in just a few more hours . . ."

I was in the middle of a contraction, so I couldn't really answer her. I remember giving her a wild-eyed look and beginning to sob convulsively. The nurse who had been assigned to my room grabbed the visitor by the arm and hauled her into a corner. While I was gathering my strength for the few minutes between contractions, they had a brief, whispered conversation. Then the visitor came back to the bed, took my hand, and said, "Okay, dear, don't think about the baby. Don't you think about that baby, just think about getting through the pain." I was already into another contraction, and once more couldn't talk. Instead I started laughing, a savage, insane sort of laugh. I was probably the most un-nerving patient that nurse ever encountered. I certainly hope so.

Every few eternities, the obstetrician on call from Harvard University Health Services would come in to see how I was doing. He'd check to see how far my cervix was dilated, tell me I was doing fine—a little slow, but fine—and go away again. I had met this doctor only once, and never since Adam was diagnosed, but I knew from Judy Trenton that none of the obstetricians at UHS agreed with my choice to continue the preg-nancy. I remembered actually wanting the doctor to come in when Katie was being born. I didn't feel that way now. It sounds harsh, but I really believed that this obstetrician would rather have delivered Adam dead than alive. He was helpful and comforting, in a pragmatic way, but my suspicions about his position on the Down syndrome issue made it hard for me to completely release myself, or Adam, to his tender mercies.

Roughly four hundred years after I'd entered the labor room, the doctor announced that I was sufficiently dilated to receive an epidural. I managed to stop yelling long enough to give my heartfelt approval for the procedure. I don't remember being even slightly discomfited when the needle was placed in my spine. Needles I could cope with. Once the anesthesia kicked in, I stopped yowling like a rabid mountain lion and began to notice my surroundings again. John held a plastic cup of water to my lips and told me I was doing great, just great. People always say this when you're in labor. It's always heartening to hear, even though everyone knows you don't have an ounce of control over what your body is doing. If there really is a way to excel at the task of labor, I defi-nitely wasn't doing it.

After the epidural kicked in, the room went very quiet. The Hispanic woman next door had been delivered of a healthy little girl. The quiet sounds of welcome and congratulation coming from her room were drowned out by the almost funereal hush in mine. After a couple more hours the obstetrician gave the order to move me into the delivery room, a place of cold, burnished metal and bright, sterile fluorescent lighting, just down the hall from the labor rooms. Before he could come in with me, John had to scrub up and put on one of the blue pajama outfits worn by the doctors. I would have made fun of the way he looked in the little shower-cap hat, but lying naked with your feet in stirrups and your body extremely distended is no position from which to be mocking anyone else's appearance. I just smiled when John came into the delivery room, and took his hand. He offered it gingerly. It was covered with little red half-moons where I'd gripped it with my fingernails, back before the epidural.

The obstetrician examined me and pronounced that it would prob-ably be only another ten minutes or so. John and I squeezed each other's hands and said nothing.

"He's crowning," the doctor told one of the nurses. "Get the others down here." The nurse ran into the hallway.

"This your first baby?" the obstetrician asked us.

We told him it was our second.

"Was your first one born with hair?" he said.

I shook my head.

"Well, this one's pretty bald, too." He smiled at me. In his face I could see compassion and regret, as well as a kind of businesslike focus. I felt a little warmer toward him, but considering my encounter with Dr. Gren-del, I kept my emotional guard up.

The metal doors swung open, and a group of five or six medical per-sonnel came through it. Most were women, dressed in a variety of white, pink, and blue uniforms, all wearing gauze masks and, of course, the obligatory shower cap. I had been told these doctors would be there. They were specialists in various areas where Adam might have trouble. As soon as he was born, they would evaluate his health and take whatever action might be necessary: heart surgery, incubation, intravenous feed-ing, and so on. Without a word, without a sound, they lined up with their backs against the wall. Their eyes above their gauze masks regarded me seriously.

It was so quiet in that room. The births of my daughters, by com-parison, were rowdy, noisy affairs, with doctors cracking jokes and John coaching me through the breathing and me occasionally mentioning that I would have preferred a quick, painless death. In the room where Adam was born, there were many more people present, but none of us made a sound. The obstetrician murmured his instructions under his breath, as though speaking loudly would have violated some private code.

I stayed silent. I could hear my own heartbeat, rapid and strong, pushed by the exertion of my anesthetized body, and by my fear. I'd forgotten the calm certainties spoken inside me back at the apartment. I was terrified. I felt as though the jury were filing in, ready to pronounce the sentence that would determine the whole of my future. The tension was unbearable. I pulled my hand away from John's, needing to face this by myself, too focused on being strong to connect with anyone. There in the center of that small but distinguished crowd, the focus of so much attention, I felt as deeply alone as I ever had in my life.

And then I remembered.

I don't know if one of them touched me again, or if they called through the silence to get my attention, or if I was the one who reached out to them, by some method I still don't understand. All I know is that suddenly I could feel the same presence, the same many presences, that had rescued me so many times while I was expecting Adam. I closed my eyes to see them better. They stood around the delivery table next to the doctors, between the instruments, over and around and through everything in that room. And they were not silent. In some wavelength beyond the range of my physical ears, I could hear the same sound that had flooded into me when I first realized I was pregnant: the singing of those great, sonorous, jubilant bells; the music of rejoicing.

"Okay," said the doctor quietly. "Give me a good strong push."

I pushed, or rather my body pushed on its own. I felt as though I were simply there for the ride. I kept my eyes closed, partly from the effort and partly because it helped me sense the silent celebration in the air around me. At that moment it was so strong, so clear, that I couldn't believe none of the doctors noticed it.

"All right," murmured the obstetrician. "There's the head."

There was no small cough, as there had been with Katie. No baby voice broke the hush. There was only that incredible sweetness, that joyful, wordless, soundless song. It was as real to me, at that moment, as if a door had been opened to another dimension, allowing me to stand for a moment on the threshold and feel that I was home.

My body tightened into another contraction, and the obstetrician pulled Adam free. As he did, the door to the bright world swung slowly, gently closed.

✐   The doctors didn't show Adam to me or John right away. The instant he was born, the medical team that had been lined up against the wall converged inward, like a football huddle with Adam at the center. They whisked him over to a small table, where they put him under a heat lamp and began to examine him.

As I tried to lift my head for a view of my baby, a rush of fear swept through me. I couldn't hear the singing as clearly anymore. I tried to feel the presence of the comforting beings who had been my friends and guardians for eight months. I could still sense them, if I concentrated, but the feeling was much fainter. Ever since Adam's conception, I had been experiencing things beyond the range of normal experience. Now that Adam was separate from me, I no longer felt like the focus of all that magic. I felt . . . normal. I felt exactly the way I wanted my son to be. It was a tremendous letdown.

I looked up at John, wanting to ask him if he could feel the angels in the room. I wanted to tell him how bereft I suddenly was, how much I wanted that strange, metaphysical connection back. But John wasn't looking at me. He had taken my hand again, but his eyes were fixed on the backs of those huddled doctors. I knew what John was hoping. I was still hoping for it, too: the sudden announcement that there had been a mistake, that Adam was fine. It never came.

Suddenly, as we watched, a long, clear, golden stream of urine arched upward, above the doctors' heads. It shifted course slightly in midair, hitting the obstetrician in the face. He jerked backward, sputtering.

"Well, his kidneys are fine," he said wryly, wiping himself with a towel.

It was the first of many, many times I would find myself swelling with pride over Adam's accomplishments.

I took a deep breath as the obstetrician came back to the table to help deliver the placenta and sew me back together. No miracle had happened. No mistakes had been made. Adam was exactly as medical science had predicted he would be. I guess I was a little sad about that. Resigned is a better word. Much worse than the confirmation of his diagnosis was my feeling that his birth had ended my sojourn into the bright place beyond the cave of my normal existence. I had been left here, in the shadow world, after only the barest glimpse of home. I didn't know the way back. I wasn't sure I could find it.

The obstetrician was almost finished with me by the time I caught my first glimpse of Adam in the flesh. My little man of earth. A doctor moved aside just as one tiny foot, about the size of a man's thumb, kicked out sideways, allowing me to see it for a fraction of a second. That was all the time I needed to see that it was not a normal foot. The big toe was set just slightly too far apart from the other four, and the two smallest toes were connected almost all the way to the tip. To most people, these abnormalities might not have been obvious, perhaps not even discernible. But I was watching for them. I knew that this was definitely the foot of a baby with Down syndrome.

I loved that foot as much as I have ever loved anything in my life.

By the time the doctors had finished their inspection, pronouncing Adam hale and hearty (except, as they delicately put it, for "his problem"), I realized that I had not been left alone after all. I was no longer the center of the high-voltage energy that had surrounded me while I was pregnant, but I was not without resources. I loved my baby. My love for him was ordinary, limited, mortal. Nothing any other mother doesn't feel. But it would do for me, because as soon as I felt it, I recognized it for what it was.

It was the way home.

33

My freshman year at Harvard, during one of my endless runs along the Charles River, I saw something glinting in the grass. It was small and pink, about the size of a pecan, and it shone in the late afternoon sunlight. I knew right away what it was, because I'd spent hours looking for things just like it during childhood hikes in the Rocky Mountains. It was a piece of rose quartz, a semiprecious stone that is supposed to symbolize compassion and friendship. When I found the chunk of quartz in Cambridge, I felt the same small thrill of delight and discovery I'd experienced as a rock-hounding child. It lay there in the emerald grass like a tiny, rosy, translucent Easter egg.

Naturally, I stopped to pick it up. As soon as I touched it I knew something was wrong. Instead of being heavy and cool and slick, like any self-respecting piece of quartz, it was very light and rather crumbly. I hefted it in my palm, looked at it more closely, and realized that this beautiful object I'd picked up was nothing more than a chunk of Styrofoam. I dropped it instantly, revolted. Instead of a lovely product of the natural world, I'd been holding a piece of pollution. I wiped my hand on my T-shirt and looked at the Styrofoam in disgust.

As I continued my run, it occurred to me that the piece of Styrofoam hadn't changed at all between the time I first saw it, when I was so drawn to its beauty, and the moment I realized what it was, and was disgusted by its ugliness. The only change was inside my head. I had assigned two different labels to that small pink object, and those labels, not the thing itself, had determined my reaction to it. This was enough to make me wonder if many of the things I reviled as ugly might not in fact be beautiful, if I might be robbing myself of beauty with my own cognitive prejudice.

I finished my run just in time to show up at one of the dormitory kitchens to work as a dining-hall grunt. My job included mopping floors and washing dishes and ladling out food to dorm residents. On the way to work, I decided to try an experiment: for that one evening, I would resist assigning any labels to my classmates as they filed through the dinner line. I would try to look at them without preconception, the way I had first looked at the Styrofoam in the grass. Of course, this is nearly impossible, but I did make an effort—for a few minutes. After that I had to stop, because I was so overcome by the beauty of every person in that dining hall that my eyes kept filling with tears. I think maybe that's one reason we screen out so much loveliness. If we saw people as they really are, the beauty would overwhelm us.

I thought about the Styrofoam quartz the first time I held Adam in my arms. Even after he was born, in the silent intensity of the doctors' examination, I was afraid of how he would look. When I caught that first glance of his foot, I was passionately relieved it did not disgust me. I was still afraid of the rest of him. I held my breath as, one by one, the doctors concluded their examinations and left. Finally, only the pediatrician was left bending over Adam. She was a short, gray-haired, fiftyish woman with a motherly voice. I watched her back as she bundled Adam into his first set of clothes. I still couldn't really see the baby.

"There we go now, little guy," said the pediatrician. At last, at long last, she picked up my baby, one hand bracing his tiny head, and brought him over to us.

He was gorgeous.

Adam was sound asleep, worn out by the process of being born. The doctor had put a little stocking hat on his head to keep him from losing body heat. The hat was striped, with a knot on one side, the tight cap of a low-ranking pirate. The head inside that hat was about the size of an orange. I could easily cup it in one hand. Adam's nose and lips and eyes were all built to scale, so tiny it was hard to believe they were real. Most babies are born looking a bit weird, their features oversized, the skin wrinkled, so that they resemble elderly relatives. Babies with Down syndrome, because their features are smaller than normal, don't look this way. They look incredibly perfect.

"Isn't he something?" said the pediatrician warmly.

John and I both jumped a little at the sound of her voice. We had been leaning forward toward Adam's face, like lovers anticipating a first kiss.

"He's not ugly," I whispered.

"Well, of course not!" said the doctor. "They're the cutest babies on earth. I have a cousin who works for Mattel. I told him they should make a Down syndrome newborn doll." She laughed. "He asked me if I'd been drinking. People don't realize."

I nodded. This doctor clearly understood about labels, how they can blind you to the beauty of things.

"Watch this," said the pediatrician. She carefully took Adam back and leaned forward, so that he was turned almost upside down. Then she lifted him upright. Adam's eyes opened, then blinked and squinted fiercely at the unaccustomed light.

"It's a reflex," she said. "It's the best way to get them to open their eyes."

Adam was already asleep again. The doctor gave him back to me, and I took him greedily. I had to force myself not to grab. The heavy, soft, warm little mound of his body inside the hospital blanket seemed to give off some kind of soothing radiation. It was highly addictive.

"Well," said the pediatrician, "I'll come up to your room later to check on him again. Right now, he looks great. You guys stay here and bond for a few minutes."

John thanked her as she left the room. I was too busy looking at Adam, drinking him in through all my senses. I loved the weight of him, the sound of his breathing, the intoxicatingly clean, sweet smell of his skin. In Adam's first portrait (taken by the hospital photographer as a service for all new babies) he resembles a cross between Mr. Magoo and a duckling, all squinty little eyes and soft blond fuzz. To me he was an infant Adonis.

"Look," said John. He reached out and picked up one of Adam's hands, which was too small to grip John's fingertip.

I stared at the hand. I will never cease to be captivated by newborn hands, and I know I'm not alone. They are so tiny, so intricate, so utterly amazing. We adults must be hardwired to react to these little hands with awe, or Lord knows we'd never do all the work required to maintain their owners. Adam's hands were even more miniature-looking than Katie's had been at her birth, because he was holding them like a grown-up; not scrunched into fists, but relaxed and open. I knew this was because of low muscle tone caused by the Down syndrome, but that was just another label. His hands, in and of themselves, were astonishingly beautiful. I stroked one with my finger. It was as soft and delicate as a wilted rose petal.

"Well," said John, after a few minutes, "here he is."

"Here he is," I agreed.

"Just like they told us."

I nodded.

"You were great, honey," John lied.

"Thanks."

"I love you." John leaned down to kiss me. Then he put one of his hands under mine and lifted Adam very gently to his face. He brushed his lips against Adam's cheek, and then his ear. The ear, I saw, was a bit too small. But it was unquestionably beautiful, a tiny, perfect, pink-and-white seashell.

"I really thought there would be a miracle," said John softly, stroking the fringe of downy white-blond hair that protruded from under Adam's pirate hat. "I really thought God would fix him."

I considered that for a minute. "Maybe he didn't need fixing," I said. "Maybe he's the only one of us who was never broken."

John looked at me. "Are you broken, sweetheart?"

"I was," I said. "Not anymore."

"Same here," said John. He paused, then gave me a smile—not his manic Harvard grin but a real smile, one that contained all the sorrow of the past months, along with the joy. "So," he said, "there's your miracle."

✎ We didn't stay at the hospital long. After that first bonding session, we couldn't seem to get any time alone together. We were sorely afflicted by a gaggle of unbearably solicitous candy stripers, who talked about everything but Down syndrome, and hordes of aspiring doctors, who talked about nothing else. Brigham and Women's is a teaching hospital, so every ten or twenty minutes another troupe of medical students, led by a full-fledged physician, would show up to see the Anomalous Baby. The students would gather round while the real doctor pointed out the symptoms of trisomy-21: the single transverse crease on the palms, the short limbs, the small facial features, the low muscle tone. I was glad that Adam was doing his part to advance medical science, but I quickly tired of his being a specimen. I took him home after barely twenty-four hours.

The only noticeable effect of his four-week prematurity was a little liver trouble. At two days old, Adam developed a slight case of jaundice, which turned his pink skin a jaunty orange. The treatment for this mild affliction involved exposing Adam's skin to direct sunlight, which helps the body synthesize vitamin D. Those first few days at home, Adam hung out in nothing but his diaper, soaking up rays from dawn to dusk. Any time a patch of sunlight came through our windows, I'd strip him down and set him on a little blanket in the light. He lay there most content-edly, his little hands gracefully limp, looking like a Chee•to-colored iguana basking in the sun. He was as lovely and amazing as any new baby, only better behaved. Katie spent hours sitting beside him, stroking his back, setting the tone for the relationship they maintain to this day.

As for me, I was doing a little basking of my own. My body was so happy not to be pregnant that I fairly floated around the apartment, buoyant with relief, the way you would if you'd suddenly recovered from an eight-month siege of stomach flu. My physical well-being almost made up for my greatly diminished sensitivity to the Bunraku pup-peteers. When I tuned into them, when I really paid attention, I could tell they were still there. But without Adam inside me, it was like looking through the proverbial glass, darkly. During the day this was enough. At night, however, it was not sufficient.

⌐ If you have ever been the primary caregiver of a newborn baby, you know how long a night can be. Adam was what we call a good baby, in that he slept a lot and only cried for food and interaction two or three times a night. However, his tiny little nostrils clogged up frequently, and he hadn't caught on to the backup strategy of breathing through his mouth, so I had to suction out his nose with a little rubber plunger every half hour or so. Thus, like most new mothers, I didn't have a lot of un-interrupted sleep to help me recover from the long ordeal of pregnancy. When you're tired, really tired, brand-new-parent tired, your view of reality can get more than slightly distorted. At 4:00 A.M. on your fifth or sixth night with virtually no sleep, the healthiest of babies can loom up before you like an immense and frightening troll who has completely taken over your life.

With Adam, I had more fears than usual to plague me during those long, long nights. The problem was that it was impossible not to fall in love with him. It is a frightening thing to love someone you know the world rejects. It makes you so terribly vulnerable. You know you will be hurt by every slight, every prejudice, every pain that will befall your beloved throughout his life. In the wee small hours, as I rocked and nursed and sang to my wee small boy, I couldn't help but worry. Will Rogers once said that he knew worrying was effective, because almost nothing he worried about ever happened. That's a cute statement, and I'm glad Will's life worked this way. But mine hasn't—at least not where Adam is concerned. Almost everything I worried about during the nights after his birth, almost every difficult thing I feared would come my way as a result of being his mother, has actually happened.

Thank God.

I was afraid Adam would slow me down, and he has. Not because he has required more care and time than a "normal" boy (he is the most helpful and least demanding of my children) but because the immediacy and joy with which he lives his life make rapacious achievement, Harvard-style, look a lot like quiet desperation. Adam has slowed me down to the point where I notice what is in front of me, its mystery and beauty, instead of thrashing my way through a maze of difficult requirements toward labels and achievements that contain no joy in themselves. Adam takes his joy straight up, in purer form than most of us can handle. He was the person who, at two years of age, spent enough time experimenting to learn that his four-month-old sister was capable of laughter, and determining exactly what would make her laugh. He is the one who goes into transports of delight over clean sheets, or packaged waffles, or batteries. He is the one who taught me to appreciate rainbows—not only in the sky but also in lawn sprinklers and dish-soap bubbles and patches of oil. He is the one who stops, and makes me stop, to smell the bushes.

I was also afraid that Adam would always be different from "normal" people. He is. If you'll cast your mind back to high school biology, you may remember that a species is defined, in part, by the number of chromosomes in every individual. Adam's extra chromosome makes him as dissimilar from me as a mule is from a donkey. He is, in ways both obvious and subtle, a different beast. I have learned that this does not mean he is simply disabled. Adam doesn't just do *less* than a "normal" child his age might; he does *different things*. He has different priorities, different tastes, different insights. Adding him to our family was like going to the pet store to buy a puppy, wanting *exactly* the kind of puppy all your friends are getting, and winding up with a kitten instead. You can spend a lot of time trying to get the kitten to fetch and bark and wag its tail, but you may also find that there is much to enjoy, to emulate, to love, about the way kittens naturally behave.

It didn't take me all that long—two or three years, I think—to stop measuring Adam's value on the barking/fetching/tail-wagging scale and notice that his "differentness" is as wonderful as I once found it frightening. His view of the world is quirky and funny and, in its own way, highly sophisticated. He is unimpressed by pretense and unmoved by convention. Don't make the mistake of thinking Adam doesn't see or understand these things. He does. He's just not interested in making them the foundation for his life. Power, wealth, prestige, and influence are not his primary concerns. I always coveted these things because I was under the illusion that they would bring me happiness; Adam goes for the happiness itself, and damn the detours. I've occasionally tried living this way since Adam came along, discarding social conformity and pursuing my heart's desires. It is as scary as the most extreme of extreme sports, but even more exhilarating.

Then, too, I was afraid that Adam would never think the way I was taught to think at Harvard. He doesn't. This was especially clear, for example, in the way Adam learned to read. He inherited our immense supply of magnetic refrigerator letters once the rest of us had stopped using them, but he didn't pick up the alphabet as Katie eventually had. Because his speech was almost completely unintelligible, I had no idea whether he was even capable of grasping the idea of written symbols representing phonetic units that can be combined to make words. Written language requires several impressive cognitive leaps, and I had no idea whether Adam would ever make even one. Nevertheless, from the time he started preschool at three, we kept running Adam through the alphabet, repeating the name of each letter, along with its major sound, thousands and thousands of times in the strained voices of tourists who believe they can overcome any language barrier by sheer volume.

It didn't work. When quizzed without prompting, Adam never recognized the letters on his own. By the time he was six I was ready to give up.

Then one day John was holding up a plastic letter and making its sound, which happened to be "EEEEEEE," when Adam suddenly perked up and said, "Wizbef!" This is the way he pronounces his sister Elizabeth's name. Naturally, John and I took this as ample cause to stay home from work and celebrate. During that day, we discovered that Adam's learning capacity went way beyond anything we expected—as long as everything he learned related directly to someone he cared about. He had absolutely no interest in, for example, "E is for egg." But E for Elizabeth— now *that* was crucial information.

In the end we all learned the alphabet this way. The symbols we had been trying to link to abstract sounds ended up as a parade of personalities: Adam first, of course, and then Billy, Caleb, Diane, Elizabeth, Francine, Grandpa . . . As we figured out how he learned, the landscape of our son's mind began to reveal itself to us. Instead of a rationally constructed structure of empirical observations, logical conclusions, and arbitrary symbols, Adam's mental world seems to be more like a huge family reunion. It is a gathering of people, all linked by Adam's affection into a complex universe of relationships and characteristics. In this world, Adam learns as fast as anyone I know. Long before he could read or write even the most basic words (or so I thought), Adam came home to tell me, in his garbled tongue, about the new boy who had just moved into his class, and who had become Adam's friend. When I couldn't understand his pronunciation of the boy's name, Adam grabbed a pencil in his stubby, grubby little-boy fingers, and wrote "Miguel Fernando de la Hoya" on a piece of paper—a piece of paper, needless to say, which I intend to frame. If I ever need a dose of Adam and he isn't around, I'll be able to look at that clumsily written name and remember what it is like to tap into an intelligence powered exclusively by love.

All of this makes Adam react in ways that are utterly different from the "Harvard responses" I had learned to venerate. While I was trying unsuccessfully to understand his pronunciation of his new friend's name, for example, Adam got laughing so hard at my wildly inaccurate guesses that he could barely breathe. Now, there are many moments when I can tell Adam is terribly frustrated by not being able to speak clearly. It bothers him. A lot. There are many times when I see the pain on his face as he struggles to communicate. These moments are intensely painful for me as well, because I know that if I were in his situation—comprehending everything around me and yet being unable to express myself—I'd want to slit my wrists. But just at the moment when Adam's frustration is most intense and I expect to see him fall into rage or despair, something changes—or rather, Adam changes something. I don't know how to describe this, except that he appears to make a conscious choice to see the situation as ridiculous. He'll take a deep breath, as though he is letting the frustration slide off his shoulders, and begin to laugh.

This is not the laughter of an idiot. It is the laughter of a person who chooses to see humor in his own discouragement, and to me it is not only intelligent but wise. In fact, I think it is wisdom in its purest form. Adam laughs at himself every day. He laughs at his own bizarre pronunciation, at the inaccurate attempts others make to understand him, at his strenuous efforts to communicate with them. He laughs as though he is being tickled over every inch of his body, finding his own plight—the plight that for me, the Harvard graduate, would be simply awful—awfully funny.

The thing is, he's right. The impromptu games of charades I play as Adam tries to talk with me are often hilarious. Because Adam is so willing to realize this, he gets everyone else to realize it, too. His laugh is so belly-deep, so apropos, so genuine, that every person within earshot ends up laughing along with him. His laughter is one of the most potent means by which he achieves his trademark effect: puncturing pomposity, posturing, self-importance, and especially intellectual pretension, wherever they occur. No indeed, Adam does not think as I was taught to think at Harvard. I hope he never will.

⌐ What my fears all boiled down to, as I sat with my tiny orange son in the days after his birth, was an underlying terror that he would destroy my own facade, the flawlessness and invulnerability I projected onto the big screen, the Great and Terrible Martha of Oz. You see, I knew all along that there wasn't one label people might apply to Adam—stupid, ugly, strange, clumsy, slow, inept—that could not, at one time or another, be justifiably applied to me. I had spent my life running from this catastrophe, and like so many other things, it caught up with me while I was expecting Adam.

In this regard, as in so many others, my worst fears have come to pass. But as they do I am learning that there is an even bigger secret, a secret I had been keeping from myself. It has been hard for me to grasp, but gradually, painfully, with the slow, small steps of a retarded child, I am coming to understand it. This has been the second phase of my education, the one that followed all those years of school. In it, I have had to unlearn virtually everything Harvard taught me about what is precious and what is garbage. I have discovered that many of the things I thought were priceless are as cheap as costume jewelry, and much of what I labeled worthless was, all the time, filled with the kind of beauty that directly nourishes my soul.

Now I think that the vast majority of us "normal" people spend our lives trashing our treasures and treasuring our trash. We bustle around trying to create the impression that we are hip, imperturbable, omniscient, in perfect control, when in fact we are awkward and scared and bewildered. The irony is that we do this to be loved, all the time remaining terrified of anyone who seems to be as perfect as we wish to be. We go around like Queen Elizabeth, bless her heart, clutching our dowdy little accessories, avoiding the slightest hint of impropriety, never showing our real feelings or touching anyone else except through glove leather. But we were dazed and confused when the openly depressed, bulimic, adulterous, rejected Princess Di was the one people really adored.

Living with Adam, loving Adam, has taught me a lot about the truth. He has taught me to look at things in themselves, not at the value a brutal and often senseless world assigns to them. As Adam's mother I have been able to see quite clearly that he is no less beautiful for being called ugly, no less wise for appearing dull, no less precious for being seen as worthless. And neither am I. Neither are you. Neither is any of us.

Of course, I haven't gone far enough in my reeducation to have left my early training completely behind me. The stupidity, the shortsightedness, the narrowness of this shadow world still hurt me from time to time. It hurt me when, three days after his birth, I carried Adam in his little front-pack to finish up my year at Harvard, and not one student or faculty member commented on the fact that he'd been born. They wouldn't even look at him. Those who had to speak to me kept their eyes resolutely fixed on my face, as though looking down a few inches at Adam's would pull them tumbling into some inescapable abyss.

That was only the beginning. Just as I feared, Adam and I have experienced mockery and judgment and exclusion, and they have all been painful. It hurts every time people look at Adam and see only the deformity of their own perceptions, instead of the beauty before their eyes. But more and more, I feel this pain not for my son but for the people who are too blind to see him. The lessons I have learned from Adam have hurt more than just about anything else I ever felt in my life. And it's been worth it, a thousand times over.

EPILOGUE

   I started dreaming about dolphins when Adam was about two, right after his younger sister was born. It was always the same dream. It began with me standing on the shore of a glassy-calm sea, watching the sun rise. Then suddenly (and no matter how many times I dreamt it, this always startled me), a dolphin broke the surface of the water in front of me, throwing itself skyward. Drops of water scattered from its fins and flanks like a shower of diamonds in the slanting light. The dolphin seemed to hang in the air for a moment, then arced downward and disappeared into the sea again.

At this point, I always experienced a feeling of intense yearning, a passionate desire to go toward the dolphin. I waded into the dream water, frightened by its depth and unfamiliarity. I am a land animal, through and through; I have always been afraid of deep water, especially in dim light. The urgency I felt to join the dolphin fought with my timidity and barely overcame it, pulling me step by frightened step into the ocean.

Then I would always look up again, out at the sea, and notice that Adam was in the water as well. He would be playing with the dolphin, his bright blond head shining like flax just above the waves. I could hear the two of them talking to each other, a strange, squealing, clicking chatter that meant nothing to me. Then the sand of the sea floor would disappear from beneath my feet and I would find myself flailing, sinking, and scared, in this world that seemed so comfortable to Adam. I wanted to go out farther—almost thought I could—but I was so terribly out of my element.

Then I would wake up.

It always took me a few minutes to come out of that dream. Even after I'd rubbed my eyes hard and climbed out of bed for a drink of water, the sense of longing that overpowered me during the dolphin dream would remain as keen as a blade. Sometimes it lasted for weeks.

Then, just when it had begun to fade from my memory, I'd go to sleep one night and have the same darn dream, all over again.

This went on for a couple of years. Every time it happened, I'd spend hours trying to figure out what it meant. I tried Freudian free association and Gestalt analysis and a booklet called *Translating the Language of Dreams* that John picked up for me at some airport newsstand. In the end, I always came back to the same conclusion: the dolphins in my dream represented . . . (drumroll, please) . . . dolphins. Porpoises, to use their technical name. Those brainy sea mammals with the endearing expressions and the highly social personalities. I was a little chagrined to have developed such a trendy passion, but there was nothing to be done about it. The dream kept coming back.

One day, when Adam was four, a neighbor of ours dropped by for a visit. When she saw Adam, she said, "I just read the most interesting article about a little boy with Down syndrome. After he was born, his mother started dreaming about dolphins. Couldn't get them off her mind."

I was so taken aback I didn't say anything at all. I had that old bristly feeling again, the one from my pregnant days.

"This woman—the mother, I mean—heard about a place in Florida where they put disabled kids in the water and let them swim with dolphins. It's some kind of therapy, I think. Would you be interested in reading the article?"

I swallowed. "Uh, yes," I said. "I think I would."

"Well, I'll just go get it now," she said.

And she did.

⌐ A few months later, when the Atlantic waters had warmed up enough to make swimming comfortable, I found myself standing on the shore of Grassy Key, Florida, helping Adam into a little yellow diving suit with pictures of Snoopy printed on it. John and the girls sat nearby, on the shore of the lagoon, talking to the animal trainer and the psychologist who ran the Dolphin Research Center. Seabirds wheeled above us, arguing with each other in raspy voices, the dawn sunlight flashing off their wings. A few feet away, watching Adam and me with eyes as brown and intelligent as the eyes of a spaniel, bobbed a dolphin by the name of Alita.

It wasn't exactly like the dream, but it was similar enough to make me unsure whether I was asleep or awake.

I slipped on my rubber diving shoes and lowered myself into the water. For just a moment, I wondered what my old classmates and professors at Harvard would think if they knew that I was paddling around a Florida lagoon with my retarded son because a recurring dream convinced me he could talk to dolphins. I didn't know, but I could make a guess.

The psychologist lowered Adam into my arms. Alita the dolphin moseyed up to me to get a closer look. I looked back at her, feeling just the way I did in my dreams.

⤶ John and I have experienced this sense of living a wonderful dream many, many times since Adam was born. The choice we made to accept him into our lives has done much more than give us a son we love to distraction. It has made risk takers of us. We are now irrationally convinced that there is little to lose by taking the road less traveled, by making decisions based on nothing but dreams, or intuition, or our hearts' desires. Since Adam came along we have quit good jobs, formed unusual relationships, undertaken projects that seemed crazy or quixotic or just plain dumb. Sometimes we succeed and sometimes we fail, but it's always a great ride.

This way of living is what took us to the Dolphin Research Center. Of course, we had a rational explanation if one should be called for. The psychologist who ran the center, Dr. David Nathanson, had a great track record helping disabled children learn to move and speak more effectively. Dr. Dave, as his patients call him, explained to me that he believes the water minimizes problems caused by lack of muscle tone, and that the dolphins are just interesting enough to distract the children from their handicaps and motivate them to learn. Right, I said. Sure. That sounds logical. But in my mind I responded, No, Dr. Dave, there's nothing logical about it. You know it and we know it. That's why we're here.

After watching Adam and the dolphins together, I was convinced that they were communicating in some method indiscernible to my mundane senses, the way the Bunraku puppeteers had communicated with me while I was pregnant. The article I got from my neighbor—the one about Dr. Dave's first young patient with Down syndrome—mentioned that the little boy had woken up one night in his bedroom, several miles inland, to grieve for a dolphin friend of his who had just died. That day in the lagoon, I could feel the same strange electric energy between Adam and the dolphins that I'd sensed around me before he was born. Go ahead and laugh, but I've been through too much to dismiss these things. I've also learned that I will probably never fully understand it. That's okay. Just being nearby is a privilege.

⌒ I swam a little way off from the shore, Adam's arm still wrapped firmly around my shoulders. We couldn't see Alita; she had disappeared into the clear green depths beneath our feet. Suddenly she shot out of the water a yard away, dousing us with a mighty splash as she belly flopped onto the surface. I nearly had a heart attack. Adam squealed with pleasure. He held his hand out, palm down, just over the water. Alita made a deft jackknife turn and came alongside, rising smoothly until her head brushed Adam's hand. I reached out to pat her as Adam grabbed her dorsal fin. Her side was as slick as a speedboat, and the muscles flexed under it like steel springs, incredibly powerful. Adam let go of me without a second glance. Alita set out for the far end of the lagoon, pulling him through the water, careful not to dunk his head. They both seemed to be laughing. Again, I had that dizzy sense of being back in my dreams. Only the chill in the water convinced me I was still awake.

What amazed me most was Adam's utter lack of fear. Before we'd come to the research center, Dr. Dave had sent us a pamphlet, warning that our child might be afraid of deep water, or large animals, or both. To prepare Adam, I'd taken him swimming once a week at a community pool. We had also visited a farm to meet some cows, which, though decidedly less streamlined than dolphins, are about the same size. Adam hated these training sessions. In the pool he clung to me like a wet mouse. The cows terrified him so much that he once used his overcoat to tie himself to a fence post, refusing to go one step closer to the pasture. I was afraid the Dolphin Research expedition would be a complete bust.

As it turned out, I was more scared than Adam. There in the waters off Grassy Key, I floundered around nervously, trying to do everything exactly right, to control this unstable, unfamiliar environment. I am, after all, still a land animal, still fond of feeling solid earth beneath my feet, afraid of deep water. The sea is beautiful but frightening, like the fluid world I entered during the time I was expecting Adam, when the rock-hard structures of Pure Reason failed me and magic came to the rescue. Maybe my life has always been as rich in mystery as it now seems. Maybe Adam merely called my attention to it. Or maybe his presence has trailed enchanting, enchanted moments into my life the way a comet trails sparks of light. Either way, I know I have far to go before I can inhabit that world without astonishment and uncertainty. It calls to me with a siren's song, but I still get scared.

That day with the dolphins, Adam wasn't scared of anything. Alita rounded the curve at the edge of the lagoon and headed back toward me, pulling him like a towrope from her fin. Adam was still laughing, the face below his golden hair radiating happiness. It is impossible to look into Adam's face when he smiles this way and not smile back. For some reason, that incredibly contagious grin reminded me of something else Albert Einstein said: that the single most important decision any of us will ever have to make is whether or not to believe that the universe is friendly. Adam appears to have made that decision.

Alita slowed down as she neared me, one mother graciously returning her baby to another. Adam swam over and seized my hand, lifting it into the air and hailing me with a triumphant shout. He didn't use words, but he didn't need any. The sound of his voice said it all. It was a cry of exultation, an expression of the pure and absolute delight Adam experiences in simply being. He put his arm around my shoulders again, but I had the feeling that instead of clinging to me for support, he was holding me up, embracing me, trying to help me trust that everything around us—the dolphins, the birds, the sun, the sky, the whole vast, blue Atlantic—was there to bring us joy.

I think he may be right.

ACKNOWLEDGMENTS

⤳ It is stunning to think about all the people who made it possible for me to write this book. The thing about a memoir is that there are so many to thank; those who helped me live through the experience, as well as those who helped me write about it.

There are a few individuals who belong in both these categories. I will never be able to fully express my love and appreciation for my husband, John Beck, who is as indispensable to me as breathing, and who stuck by me through the whole damn thing. Katie Beck, though only eighteen months old at the time this story began and only twelve now, cared for me as best she could while I produced her brother and this book. (I hope it will serve as a pre-written confession to any therapist who may someday end up helping Katie process her childhood traumas.) Sibyl Johnston, brilliant writer, loyal friend, and poorly disguised angel of mercy, also has my endless gratitude, as does her husband, Charles Inouye. My cousin Lydia Nibley brought an unexpected ray of hope and delight into one of the worst periods of my life. She and her sister Sylvia Nibley have continued to dazzle me with their love and support.

Other people who saved my life while I was expecting Adam include my parents, Hugh and Phyllis Nibley, and John's parents, Jay Beck and his late wife, Faye. My sisters—Christina Mincek, Rebecca Nibley, and Zina Petersen—provided endless physical and emotional help, as did my brother Paul and his wife, Bronia. On the Harvard front, John and I received still more kindness from friends like Anne and Kenneth Morrell, Diane and Lant Pritchett, and other friends from the graduate-student community. Faculty members who were particularly thoughtful and supportive include Will Reimann, Dr. Annemette Sørensen, Dr. Lenore Weitzman, Professor Aage Sørensen, Professor Ezra Vogel, and Professor John Kotter. Bev Douhan of the Department of Sociology was also unfailingly generous with her time and compassionate advice. Dr. Walter

Ames and Mark Fuller were especially crucial in helping John continue his career despite the complications caused by my poor health and Adam's diagnosis. They may never know how deeply I appreciate them.

A whole new division of helpers came on the scene once I had finished living the story and started writing it. My third child, Lizzie, was on the way. From the moment Adam first discovered how to make her laugh, when she was still so small her head fit in the palm of my hand, Lizzie has been his best friend. Like Katie and Adam, she has forgiven my many parental weaknesses and brought me enormous happiness. Other than John, Dr. Ruth Killpack was the person who most consistently convinced me my story was worth recounting. Her love and expertise helped me find my voice. My fellow travelers Connie, Anne, Olga, Marcy, Melanie, Pam, and Linda all cheered me on in my writing and my life, and I adore them as well. Silja Allen and Patricia Holland helped me make sense of my own experiences so that I could write about them with something approaching clarity. Dawn Swanson gave me crucial input and camaraderie soon after we relocated to Phoenix. Annette Rogers was my first (informal) editor. Her patience and constructive criticism would have made her my sworn friend, even if she hadn't been one already.

After the first version of *Expecting Adam* was finished, Susan Schulman, my agent, read it and took me in off the street. She provided feedback, encouragement, advice, and a lot of hard work to get the book published—and was great fun to talk to, besides. I'm grateful for the many people at Times Books who assisted in the publication process: John Rambow, Peter Bernstein, Mary Beth Roche, Carie Freimuth, and Nancy Inglis, to name a few. Special love and thanks to my amazing editor, Betsy Rapoport, whose intelligence and sensitivity set the right course for this book, and whose friendship gave me the courage to follow it.

Finally, I want to thank Karen Gerdes, whose constant wisdom, compassion, and clarity of vision have healed so many wounds and brought so many hopes to fruition. Seeing all these people listed on one page is truly overwhelming. If you'll excuse me, I think I'll lie down and cry for a while.

AUTHOR'S NOTE

꙳ This is a work of nonfiction, meaning that it contains a rigorously factual account of real events, along with the occasional bald-faced lie about the people involved in them. Allow me to explain.

In writing *Expecting Adam*, I made a scrupulous effort to report exactly what happened to me during my second pregnancy. One of my reasons for putting it all down in the first place was to fix the details of my experience on paper so that my memory wouldn't distort them over time. This was intensely important to me, since I was recording events I myself found incredible, events that ultimately changed the way I see the world. Moreover, I knew that if the book ever got published, I would promptly achieve the status of Certified Fruit Bat among all my academic friends and acquaintances. If I was to be accused of exaggeration or flat-out invention, I wanted to be absolutely sure these accusations were ungrounded.

I have had plenty of training in recording "just the facts." My schooling as a Harvard-pedigreed sociologist involved being violently attacked (not physically, but close) whenever my accounts of events were sloppy, inflated, or poorly substantiated. Over the years, I've made habits out of taking exhaustive notes, recording interviews, and rechecking my own interpretation of events against other people's perceptions. I spent thousands of hours before writing my first book, *Breaking Point*, sifting through every bit of data to make sure I could confirm it factually. I have done the same thing here.

To assist my memory as I wrote *Expecting Adam*, I had a voluminous journal that I'd kept during my pregnancy. It was packed with every minuscule tidbit of my thought and experience, including the gist—and often the exact words—of important conversations. For years I kept reminding myself to burn this journal, until I finally realized that any sane person would prefer being deep-fried to actually reading the thing. It survived to become the main information source for this book. John's experience was partially available to me through the journal and the Seeing Thing (as I explain in this book), but I also forced him to slog through hours of reminiscing and fact checking to ensure that I'd captured his experiences fairly and accurately. When the manuscript was finished, I called the friends I'd portrayed in it to make sure my memories squared with theirs.

As it turned out, my quest for accuracy became something of a problem. I found that when I was writing about real people in a nonfiction format, I ran a considerable risk of causing them distress, often by revealing things about them that seem completely innocuous to me. I have therefore changed the names and identifying characteristics of many people described in these pages; I have indicated all of these disguises in the text. My objective is to protect the privacy of both dear friends and those whose unflattering words and actions (which appear unaltered) speak for themselves.

You are therefore holding a book that recounts (1) a lot of ordinary, believable stuff involving people you'll never be able to pick out of a police lineup, although I believe some of them belong there; and (2) some really weird, unbelievable stuff, all of which is recorded exactly as it happened. In other words, the harder something is to believe, the truer it is likely to be. The more I think about it, the more this seems to be the way things are with life in general.